HUMAN DEVELOPMENT

Experiences of North East India

HUMAN DEVELOPMENT
Experiences of North East India

Editors
Kiran Sankar Chakraborty
Gurudas Das

AKANSHA PUBLISHING HOUSE
New Delhi - 110 002

AKANSHA PUBLISHING HOUSE
4649-B/21, Ansari Road
Darya Ganj, New Delhi - 110 002
Ph.: 23263193/9811582579
Fax: 011-23263193
Email: ektabooks@yahoo.com

Human Development: Experiences of North East India

First Published 2007
ISBN 81-8370-039-X

PRINTED IN INDIA

Published by M.P. Misra for Akansha Publishing House, New Delhi and Printed at Aryan Enterprises, Delhi

PREFACE

Human development is a powerful concept than conventional measure of gross national product (GNP) in understanding human well being. With the rejection of "trickle down hypothesis", rising disillusion with assumed positive association between growth and well-being, new insights gained in the relationship between growth and equity that nullifies the claim of negative relationship at least at early stage of growth, the exploration of the capability approach towards development and the emergence of the new growth theories that focus on the role of the human factor in economic growth—all have brought a sharp focus on the human development as a necessary condition for sustainable growth.

Human development can be viewed as a process of enlarging people's choices. Increase in per capita income is one of the main means of expanding choices and well being. Enhancing people's capabilities is equally important for judging the well-being of mankind. Capabilities like knowledge, health, self-respect and ability to participate actively in community life enhances people's choices to lead the lives they value. Besides material needs, people also value their freedom, e.g., freedom of movement, freedom of speech and freedom from oppression, violence and exploitation. People also need a sense of purpose in their life and a sense of empowerment. People also prefer to protect their culture and maintain social cohesion. These social and cultural capitals are no less important for the well-being of man. Money can hardly buy them. They need to be created through collective actions and transmitted inter-generationally. The increasing acceptance of this perspective has led to the global rethinking as to how to convert the free market led extreme individualistic social development into more socially responsible and communitarian form of development. People's choices will be enlarged only when they acquire critical capabilities like knowledge and health. Although acquisition of capabilities have their own intrinsic value, it is not mere acquisition of human capabilities that will enhance human development unless those acquired capabilities are used for higher attainment of income and other statuses that make their life more meaningful and worthy. Thus, the discourse of human development has both intrinsic as well as instrumental value.

It is needless to mention that human development is also a prerequisite for sustained and faster economic growth. Expansion of human capabilities leads to skill formation and raises the productivity of the workforce. Increase in productivity enables the workers to produce more without additional costs. Production becomes competitive and hence widens market accessibility. Entrepreneurship grows and innovations take place. Skilled workforce attracts foreign direct investments in the economy. Moreover, with the rising level of education, the whole production process benefits from "positive externalities" and causes a rise in the efficiency of all factors of production. The rise in the level of education of the workforce offsets, to a significant extent, the decreasing marginal returns to capital. In fact, the modern economic growth largely related with the pace of innovation. The higher the quality of human development, the faster is the pace of innovation in an economy as it is endowed with highly educated manpower required for carrying out research and development activities and skilled workforce to put the results into practice

Thus, human development acts as the driving force of all economic growth. The forces of economic growth and human development reinforce each other and take both the economy and the people forward. An understanding of this dynamic relationship between these two has led to the idea of the "people centered development strategy" for the developing countries in recent times as opposed to "capital centered development strategies" of the 1950s.

Contributions in this volume have attempted to focus on the different dimensions of the discourse on economic growth and human development. Attempts have also been made to assess the status and condition of human development in the states of North East India.

The book is a collection of research papers contributed by scholars of various organisations in North-East India. There are 15 papers in the book focussing upon the issues associated with human development in north-eastern region of India. Out of which 13 were presented in a national seminar on "Human Resource Development in North-East India" at Agartala held on 18-19 September, 2004. The seminar was organised by Economic Science Society of Tripura (ESSOT), a renowned academic organisation of the state. We owe a great deal to the Economic Science Society of Tripura for their consent to publish the papers. Two papers of the volume (chapter 8 and 13) were published in the Journal of North-East India Council for Social Science Research, Shillong (Vol. 29 No. 2 October, 2005). We are thankful to NEICSSR for its consent to incorporate these two papers in this volume.

We express our deep sense of gratitude to the contributors. We also acknowledge our gratitude to Mr. Bhupal Chandra Sinha, General Secretary, ESSOT and Dr. Haradhan Debnath, Reader, School of Management, Tripura University, for their constant support and encouragement.

Finally we express our indebtedness to Mr. M.P. Misra of Akansha Publishing House, New Delhi, for taking all pains for publishing this book.

Agartala
August 15, 2006

Kiran Sankar Chakraborty
Gurudas Das

Contents

List of Tables

List of Flow Charts

List of Boxes

Contributors

Chakraborty, Gorky: Fellow, Department of Economics, Dibrugarh University, Dibrugarh, Assam

Chakraborty, K.S.: Regional Director, IGNOU Regional Centre, Agartala

Das, Anil Kumar: Asstt. Profesor Department Statistics, MBB College, Agartala

Das, Gurudas: Head, Department of Humanities and Social Sciences, National Institute of Technology, Silchar-788012

Datta, Anup Kumar: Asstt. Profesor Department of Economics, BBM College, Agartala

De, Utpal Kumar: Reader, Department of Economics, NEHU, Shillong.

Dutta, Rajesh: Lecturer, Department of Economics, St. Edmund's College, Shillong.

Dutta, Subhendu: Department of Economics, Pubic College of Commerce, Dimapur, Nagaland.

Hazarika, Padmalochan: Faculty Member, Department of Commerce, Guwahati University, Assam.

Roy, Hiranmoy: Lecturer, Department of Economics, Karimganj College, Assam

Ray, Santanu: Department of Economics, Mizoram University, Aizwal.

Sarkar, Abhijit: Asstt. Profesor, Department of Economics, R.K.Mahavidyalaya, Kailshahar

Sengupta, Keya: Professor, Department of Economics, Assam University, Silchar

Singh, K. Gyanendra: Department of Economics, NEHU, Shillong.

Tluanga, R. Lalnun: Reader, Department of Economics, Aizwal North College, Mizoram.

Section I
Globalisation, Social Capital, Environment and Human Development

1

GLOBALIZATION AND HUMAN DEVELOPMENT: IS THERE ANY TRADE OFF ?

– Gurudas Das

Does globalization lead to human development? Are the processes of globalization and human development complementary to each other? Or, does any trade off exist between them? In fact, if globalization is viewed as a means and human development as an end, then, the apparent contradiction between them becomes readily evident. While globalization is capital centered, human development is people centered. While the former calls for strengthening the forces of market, the achievement of the latter calls for effective state intervention. While the advocates of globalization prescribe for the reduction of public expenditure in social sectors like education, health care, old age pension, etc., the proponents of human development argue in favour of extension of such services under public sector.

This apparent contradiction gives way to seeming complementarity when globalization is viewed as means to achieve economic growth without which human development is hard to come by. Moreover, while human development aims at expanding the human capabilities and widening the choices; globalization, by expanding the economic opportunities, enables the nations to realize the goals of human development. However, as it has already been observed, this link between economic growth and human development by no means automatic

(HDR:1990). Hence, nations need to strike a balance between the agenda of globalization and human development.

Needless to say that this complementarity view is uncritical of the positive link between globalization and economic development. It is not that all the countries have been benefited while embracing globalization. While globalization worked in Asia, it failed in Africa, Latin America and Central Europe. Even where it has worked, it is not that all the sections of the society and all the sectors in an economy have been benefited in equal proportions. The modern sectors and the work force engaged in them have been the gainer while the traditional sectors and people engaged in them have been the looser. This paper intends to focus on the interlinkages between the twin processes of globalization and human development. In that, it focuses on the positive aspects of globalization and then argues as to how it can be tamed for the enhancement of human development particularly in the developing countries.

Human Development and Economic Growth: The Two-Way Linkages

Human development is often defined as a process of enlarging people's choices (HDR: 1990). People's choices will be enlarged only when they acquire critical capabilities like knowledge and health. It is not mere acquisition of human capabilities that will enhance human development unless those acquired capabilities are used for higher attainment of income and other statuses that make their life more meaningful and worthy. Thus, for enhancing the human capabilities massive investment in education and health is called for. The question is: where from this investment will come. Certainly, both the private and public sector have a role to play in this regards. The problem is: if these services are catered only by the private sector, the price may be out of the reach of the poor who constitute the majority in most of the developing countries. And hence, dependence on the market for providing these services will tantamount to denying them to the vast majority. This, instead of enhancing, will slowdown the progress of human development. Thus, two options are available: either raise the real income per capita to such a level so that people can afford them at market price or provide them at subsidized rates or free of cost across the board through public spending so that people can have easy and costless access to these services. As economic growth takes off and people's purchasing power increases, the domain of the public expenditure on social sectors may gradually be substituted by private initiatives. Without sustained economic growth, it becomes difficult for the state to make sustained investment in social sectors. Thus, without economic growth state can only make limited investments in social sectors and private sector will hardly find it profitable to invest in the areas of education and health. However, this portrays one side of the story. The other side involves the use of the acquired human capabilities. This requires the expansion of economic opportunities so that people can choose their livelihood and make the best use of their capabilities. This is certainly not possible unless the economy grows and provides a space to all those who want to grow. Economic growth, therefore, is a *sine qua non* for the sustained human development.

Human development is also a prerequisite for sustained and faster economic growth. Expansion of human capabilities leads to skill formation and raises the productivity of the workforce. Increase in productivity enables the workers to produce more without additional costs. Production becomes competitive and hence widens market accessibility. Entrepreneurship grows and innovations take place. Skilled workforce attracts foreign direct investments in the economy. Moreover, with the rising level of education, the whole production process benefits from "positive externalities" and causes a rise in the efficiency of all factors of production. The rise in the level of education of the workforce offsets, to a significant extent, the decreasing marginal returns to capital (HDR: 1996). In fact, the modern economic growth largely related with the pace of innovation. The higher the quality of human development, the faster is the pace of innovation in an economy as it is endowed with highly educated manpower required for carrying out research and development activities and skilled workforce to put the results into practice. A World Bank study of 192 countries has established that only 16 per cent of growth is explained by physical capital, 20 per cent by natural capital and rest 64 per cent by human and social capital (HDR:1996).

It is worth to mention here the four-fold classification of the global experiences relating to economic growth and human development made by the UNDP (HDR:1996).

First, countries having higher human development but slower economic growth in one decade either increased economic growth in the next or experienced poor economic growth and slow human development. This shows that if human development is not matched with economic growth, it is difficult to sustain in the long run.

Second, countries having fast economic growth but slow human development have experienced economic growth petering out in the long run.

Third, countries having both fast economic growth and human development experienced mutually reinforcing virtuous circle. In this case, both economic growth and human development are sustainable.

Fourth, countries having both slow economic growth and human development experienced mutually stifling growth and human development.

Thus, human development acts as the driving force of all economic growth. The forces of economic growth and human development reinforce each other and take both the economy and the people forward. An understanding of this dynamic relationship between these two has led to the idea of the "people centered development strategy" for the developing countries in recent times as opposed to "capital centered development strategies" of the 1950s.

Does Globalization lead to economic growth?

The process of globalization, viewed in terms of integration of the national economies with the global economy by way of adopting uniform legal framework, has both costs and benefits. It has created both opportunities and vulnerabilities. Besides the developed countries, some developing countries, mostly in Asia, like China, Malaysia, South Korea, Singapore, India, Indonesia, Mauritius, Chile, Poland, the Dominic Republic, Costa Rica, Botswana, and Turkey have gained in terms of economic growth, many in Africa, Latin America and Eastern Europe have failed to reap any benefit of globalization.

Liberalization and deregulation of national markets, reduction in tariff and expansion of trade, fast growth of information technology and its impact on the reduction of costs and raising the productivity, the tertiary revolution, free mobility of global capital and the transformation from manufacturing to knowledge-based economy—all have released tremendous opportunities before the nations. With the growth of global competition, MNCs/TNCs are increasingly relocating manufacturing activities from high wage locations to low wage locations. As a result, manufacturing process, instead of vertical integration, is experiencing some sort of deverticalization.

The heightened competition brought about by Globalization has made a deep impact in corporate strategies of firms particularly of the MNCs/TNCs . All most in every sphere of industrial production ranging from automobile to electronics—corporate houses are embracing deverticalization either through the establishment of subsidiaries or through subcontracting or outsourcing. Firms are increasingly moving out of "Chandlerian Prototype" to "Wintelist" Prototype. Original Equipment Manufacturers (OEM) are no longer aiming at vertical integration of manufacturing process, rather to cope up with stiff competition, they prefer to fragmentation of production in order to relocate manufacturing in low wage locations. Migration of industrial activities from high wage locations to low wage locations has been one of the distinct trends that has become prominent since early 1990's.

As per the globalization-driven corporate strategy, the OEM's concentrate on "core competence" consisting mainly of R&D, product designing, assembling, sales, marketing and after sales services, while the job of manufacturing is either outsourced to suppliers or sub-contracted to other firms operating particularly in low-wage locations.

This trend of fragmentation, deverticalization and relocation of manufacturing production process has led manufacturing actives to shift form high wage economics of USA and Western Europe to countries in Eastern Europe, China and newly industrialized nations in South East Asia. The relocation of labour-intensive industries from high wage to low wage locations is quite vivid. For example, employment figures of the German apparel industries declined from 185,510 in 1989 to 48,362 in September 2003, manufacturing migrated, via outsourcing, to low-cost regions. However, although the apparel industries in Germany are constantly shrinking both with regard to employment and number of companies, this loss is compensated by gains made in other areas.

Unlike apparel industry, the German automobile industry is the winner of globalization. Although it has also underwent production fragmentation and relocation (particularly in Eastern European countries like Czech Republic, Hungary, Slovakia and Poland), the loss of jobs at home is not very substantial. The Volkswagen, the leading German car maker, has pushed its employment figurer abroad from 95000 in 1990 to 159000 in 2000 leading to slight decline of jobs at home. Thus, the automobile industry in Germany shows a picture where the negative impact of globalization regarding several sub sector and particular employee groups is compensated by positive effects in other sub sectors and employee groups, whereas this could not be achieved in the German apparel industry.

Like the apparel and automobile industries, electronics firms of Western Europe like Siemens, Alcatel, Philip's have also shifted a large chunk of their manufacturing bases to Eastern European countries.

While the West European firms control the more demanding and sophisticated tasks like process development, industrialization of the product, prototyping, production planning and ramp-up of production, they subcontract standardized manufacturing activities to low wage locations in Eastern Europe. Thus, Eastern European countries are becoming the production house that caters the customer demands of the west. Geographical and cultural proximity appear to be the prime causes for the migration of Western firms to East instead of other low-wage locations elsewhere.

Besides Eastern European countries, China has already emerged as the workshop of the world. Low-wage, high-class infrastructure, high growth rate and huge internal market -- are some of the reasons that make China attractive for relocation and foreign direct investment. Huge internal demand has given a great boost to Chinese automobile industries. Almost all the global players have rushed to China with major investment projects. China Industrial Development Report on the Auto Industry in China 2003 observed that by next 10 to 15 years, China would become the largest auto market in the world. What is more important is the export of Chinese made auto parts. The American manufacturers are particularly keen to benefit from the low cost condition in China. General motors and Ford are pursuing their suppliers to open factories in China. In 2003, new automotive factories have been built in 23 provinces and cities in China. A report of Boston Consulting Group has estimated a cost advantage of 10 to 20 percent for large established car venture in China and up to 40 percent for smaller operators.

Like the auto industries, China has emerged as the world largest base for electronic parts. While the electronic production in emerging market were nearly double – from US $65 billion in 2001 to US $125 billion by 2005, China will have the lion share of this growth, 77 percent. International Finance Corporation and Boot Allen Hamilton have predicted an increase of Chinese share in global electronic production from 8 percent to 14 percent. China has already become the leading producer of DVD-Rom drives, DVD players, Desktop personal computer, colour television and mobile phones.

Besides, Eastern Europe and China, the process of fragmentation and relocation of industrial process has also led to the migration of global manufacturing companies to countries in South East Asia. Now the question is: why do firms relocate in certain low-wage location bypassing other such locations? Apart from the main centers of relocation already mentioned, there are many more low-wage locations in Asia, Africa and Latin America, why these locations are not chosen? One of the plausible explanations is: mere low-wage alone does not determine the site for relocation. Size of the internal market, existing infrastructural facilities, availability of skill labour force and most importantly, capacity of the local supplier to deliver goods in time – all are taken into consideration in arriving at a decision on the site of relocation.

Apart from manufacturing, service outsourcing has become another major trend of globalization. For becoming a hub of service providing activities, no huge investment in infrastructure is required. Human resource plays the key role. India has become the most favoured destination for IT enable services largely due to the availability of technical manpower.

Thus, globalization has fueled the demand for high skilled jobs while the demand for unskilled jobs is on the wane. The sunrise sectors include the information technology enable services, biotechnology, electronic and telecommunication industry, analytical instruments, pharmaceuticals, automobile, banking and insurance, etc. while most of the traditional manufacturing activities are experiencing sun set syndrome. This technology and market led globalization is driving the global economy towards these sunrise sectors that are experiencing fast growth. Firms and the workforce associated with these sectors are gaining in terms of growth in income.

Integrating with the global economy *per se* is no guarantee for economic growth. Countries like Madagascar, Niger, the Russian Federation, Tajikistan, Cameroon, Venezuela and sub-Saharan Africa are not less integrated but they have shown little growth (HRD:1999). With falling international prices, primary producing countries are finding it hard even to maintain their previous growth rates.

Countries that could gain from globalization differ in terms of quality of growth. Many countries suffer from jobless growth where enough employment opportunities have not been created. For a pro-people growth, the rate of job creation should be higher than the rate of growth of labour force. The use of capital-intensive technology has led to the increase in productivity but created very little employment in the economy. In all most all the countries, the wage gap between the skilled and unskilled labour has been widened.

Globalization has resulted into both horizontal inequality across regions and vertical inequality within the nations. Flexible labour laws and environmental standards adopted by many countries in order to attract foreign direct investment have led to the casualisation of jobs, increase work time, job insecurity, and environmental degradation.

Globalization and Human Development

Globalization of IMF-WB-WTO variety coached in neo-liberal thoughts aims at increasing efficiency and trade led growth. Liberalization, privatization and market fundamentalism constitute the building blocks of structural adjustment programmes. Fund-Bank-Organization conditionalities call for capital market liberalization, reduction in the state activism in terms of public expenditure in social sectors, subsidy for production and consumption, expenditure relating to social security measures, investment for the removal of horizontal and vertical inequalities and providing job security through the formulation of labour laws, privatization of public assets and reduction in tariffs. All these are aimed to squeeze the state initiatives and to make the state subservient to market forces. Thus, this variety of globalization is all about the triumph of markets over governments (Steger: 2004).

However, the experiences of the countries who could gain from globalization prove to be otherwise. The experiences of China, India, Malaysia, Republic of Korea, Indonesia, Poland, Botswana—all show that globalization worked in them not because of unfettered operation of the market forces but because of the active patronage of the governments in managing the globalization (Stiglitz:2002). Adoption of labour intensive technology in China and South East Asian countries has helped in establishing a link between economic growth and employment opportunities making globalization work for the people at large, huge public sector investment in creating infrastructure in them has made them attractive for foreign direct investment. In all these countries governments made substantial investment in education and health care in order to improve human resource quality so that people could acquire the capabilities needed to make use of the opportunities arising out of the operation of the forces of globalization. South East Asian countries have put an egalitarian income distribution mechanism in place that automatically takes care of vertical income inequality impact of growth. India has not made its capital market fully convertible and hence could survive from the contagion effect of South East Asian currency crisis.

While the shift towards knowledge base economy necessitates

a huge investment on the part of the state to educate and train the labour force in that direction so that people could acquire the necessary skills demanded by the market, the prescription of the Fund-Bank-Organization to undermine the role of the state just works in opposite direction. This is more true in case of the countries where income distribution is skewed, human development is low, growth is stagnated and wide differences exist between the required and achieved human capabilities. Not only has the international regulatory framework restrained governments for undertaking social sector expenditure, reduction of tariff across the board, waiver of corporate tax, tax incentives offered to business and industries, establishment of tax free export processing zones— all have also squeezed the government exchequer and crippled them. Countries that have followed Fund-Bank-Organization prescription for economic growth could hardly succeed in generating growth while countries that have followed policies independent of them could reap the benefits of globalization to certain extent.

The process of globalization as such does not stand on the way of human development. State led globalization *a la* China, Malaysia, India, Poland, Botswana has rather helped to achieve higher growth, reduction of poverty, creation of jobs, as against Fund-Bank-Organization guided market led globalization. Competitive markets may help in increasing efficiency but also creates inequality, concentration of wealth, act as disincentives for non-market care giving services which are otherwise essential for the well being of mankind.

The "one-size-fits-all" approach of the international institutes provides little room to the nations having diverse socio-political and economic conditions to sequence and adjust their respective economies with the process of globalization. Withdrawal of the governments from social sector services before the markets in them could develop has either slowed down or reversed human development in many countries. Instead of gradual replacement of public services by private initiatives, the insistence of the international agencies to substitute government by market overnight has led to the collapse of many a social service in the developing countries. As a result, the quality of life of the poor people in countries like the Russian Federation, Eastern European, Sub-Saharan Africa and Latin America has deteriorated.

Thus, there exists a trade off between the Fund-Bank-Organization guided market led globalization and human development. Until the global governance focuses on the priorities of human development, globalization is hard to sustain. Market efficiency and global competition are only means to achieve economic growth. But economic growth cannot be an end in itself. It is again a means to achieve the goal of human well being. A simultaneous progress in economic growth and human development can only release the necessary reinforcing forces that will make both globalization and human well being sustainable in the long run. For this to happen, market is not any substitute for the community and government. Either the globalizers have to reorient and restructure the focus of globalization or they have to invent an alternative path that suits their respective specificities in order to make globalization work for their people in the long run.

REFERENCES

Human Development Report, 1990, UNDP, OUP, New York.

Human Development Report, 1991, UNDP, OUP, New York.

Human Development Report, 1996, UNDP, OUP, New York.

Human Development Report, 1999, UNDP, OUP, New York.

Steger, Manfred B., 2004, (first Indian reprint), *Globalization: The New Market Ideology*, Rawat Publications, Jaipur.

Stiglitz, Joseph E., 2002, *Globalization and its Discontents*, Penguin Books, New Delhi.

2

ROLE OF HUMAN AND SOCIAL CAPITAL IN ECONOMIC DEVELOPMENT

– *Rajesh Dutta*

Issues & Concerns

As time has progressed, incalculable appreciable and imperceptible changes have swept across all spheres of the human life, as well as the natural / physical environment. As the pace of these changes varied across the globe, perceptive minds analysed and justified for the dissimilarities and directly and /or indirectly suggested several remedial measures. Suffice to say that no single factor can be factored out because with the proliferation of social complexities, the dimension and the density of indicators have also compounded. In the quest to make sense of a variety of 'what, why and how' questions in any discipline, newer ones are continuously surfacing and to be truly convincing and articulate one has to traverse across multiple disciplines.

The gist of development is an all encompassing one and while the debate regarding what is economic growth and economic development appears settled, the process by which the alterations should come forth are still mired in a labyrinth since a multitude of variables must be taken into consideration. The choice of appropriate indicators requires adequate justification over a period of time and across nations in different societies.

The general consensus on development is on human well-being (both economic and general well-being). The employment of a range of indicators to capture economic and non-economic attainments (or alternatively, the extent of deprivations) has evolved some sort of a yardstick to measure the standard of living. Many of the outcomes are either desirable in themselves or because they have an important role to play in enhancing the future possibilities for people. If by the process of development we seek to expand human capabilities by the provision of choices/ options to help people lead the kind of life that they desire, then it must be complemented by the opening up as well as the expansion of economic opportunities and the creation of social conditions which will facilitate the use of those opportunities [Dreze & Sen (1998), pp.5-7]. In this connection while the range of indicators provide some guidance for developmental interventions for achieving desirable outcomes, the complex interaction of different forces and factors that truly shape the outcomes, cannot be ignored. The process of development has never been automatic and it is progressively being realised that the 3 forms of capital (natural, physical and human) only partially determine the growth process, because they overlook the process of interactions between economic agents and how they organise themselves to promote growth and development [Grootaert (1998), pp. 1]. Apparent from a number of studies is that several intangible forces, shaped by historical, cultural, social and political factors, critically affect developmental outcomes.

This chapter makes no pretence of presenting anything new or anything substantial. It simply reviews and reassesses some existing literature to draw attention to the following:

(a) The importance of investing in humans – via investments in education and health

(b) Nurturing the intangible forces to make development consequential and sustainable – by giving due importance to Social Capital

(c) Pro – active role of various institutions and the State – or the policy implications

Human Capital - Meaning & Significance

People play a vital role as agents of change in the development process and they are also the beneficiaries. But, the scale of participation and the distribution of the benefits are not always equitable. People must therefore possess certain capabilities and virtues as agents and harbingers of change and such acceptance is essentially the result of an array of empirical studies undertaken over the last four decades. The idea of human capital came into existence in the early 1960s when particular attention was devoted to the quality of labour, the level of education and training in the workforce [OECD (2001), pp17]. Human capital is now defined as "the knowledge, skills, competence and attitudes embodied in individuals that facilitate the creation of personal, social and economic well-being" [Ibid pp18]. It has been established that the quality of human capital benefits beyond the individual and spills over to the society as well. A broader notion of human capital includes not only the acquired cognitive but also the non-cognitive skills which can be developed in the contexts of (i) learning within family (ii) formal education and training (iii) workplace training and (iv) informal learning on-the-job and in daily and civic participation [Ibid]. Besides, human capital is also developed in specific cultural settings [Ibid] and the role of social networks and norms in nurturing a culture of learning throughout the entire lifespan of people is considered important [Ibid pp20]. High levels of social engagements and trust open up opportunities for both formal and informal learning and the levels of civic participation is strongly related to the levels of initial education, continuing education and learning [Ibid pp24].

The Influence of Human Capital

The impact of education and human capital on economic well being and general well being is well documented. Although the manifold benefits arising from the spill over and positive externalities are difficult to accurately estimate and measure, micro-level research demonstrates a positive relation between education, earnings and employment. For instance, an additional year of education, on an average, has led to higher earnings in the range of 5 – 15 per cent [Krueger and Lindahl (1999) in OECD (2001), pp28]. Further, labour market earnings show a positive co-relation between higher levels of adult literacy and knowledge intensity of occupations [Raudenbush and Kasim (1998) in OECD (2001), pp28].

At the macro-level, it has been difficult to trace the role of human capital on growth. Comparisons between developing and developed countries attempted by some studies have not been entirely convincing because the factors determining growth vary across countries. Inconclusive answers, though, point to the poor quality of data and the practical difficulties in identifying the manner that human capital affects the growth process. But recent studies confirm more a dynamic impact of human capital on economic growth. Taking the OECD countries as a whole, an extra year of full education (estimated to increase human capital by 10 %) has shown an increase in per capita output by about 6 per cent [OECD 2001, pp 31].

There is evidence of the impact of human capital on other aspects of human well-being affecting the quality of life. Education and learning can indirectly bring forth many social benefits. A clear benefit of education is on health. Better educated people were found to have healthier habits and lifestyles because educated people were in a better position to identify health related information and use this information to realize behaviour favourable to better health [Kenkel (1991) in OECD (2001), pp33].

The educational level of one generation has positive effects on the next generation and also on civic participation. Education helps lower crime rates by reducing anti- social behaviour and also improves subjective well-being and happiness.

To reiterate, it has been well documented that education, training and learning have helped build human capital and provide the base for economic growth (provided that opportunities exist) through greater social cohesion. However, as mentioned earlier, human capital can only partially determine the growth process. The process and the degree of interactions between economic agents and how they organise themselves to promote growth and development, necessitates closer scrutiny and re-examination. In doing so we are purposefully guided toward another notion viz. Social Capital presently attracting the attention of many.

Social Capital - Meaning & Significance

The realisation that non- economic factors play an equally, if not more, essential role in any developmental process has led to investigations of their specifics. In the course of these pursuits the concept of Social Capital materialized. The World Bank's Social Capital website (http://www.worldbank.org/poverty/scapital/) defines social capital as "*the institutions, relationship, and norms that shape quality and quantity of a society's social interactions.*" It highlights the importance of 'horizontal' and 'vertical' associations and states that the "the broadest and most encompassing view of social capital includes the social and political environment that shapes social structure and enables norms to develop". The social capital concept is not new [for literature reviews refer to Woolcock (1998) & OECD (2001)]. Durkheim, Weber and Marx were deeply influenced by the economic issues and debates of their period and what is now termed as 'social capital' were also their primary concerns [Swedberg (1987)]. But, the role of norms and institutions in explaining economic life were suppressed for much of the 19th century and classical political economists developed social science along the path of Adam Smith's *The Wealth of Nations* rather than his *The Theory of Moral Sentiments* [Collins (1994) in Woolcock (1998) pp 160].

Social capital is profusely defined and used. In the west, the notion has been largely used to study the nature of democracy and the democratic functioning of institutions. In developing countries, the term has been utilised to reveal its importance in augmenting development. Social interactions among economic agents play a vital role in encouraging the growth process and the nature and magnitude of these interactions are dependent on several factors. The strength of social connectedness and social cohesion are crucial for any development outcome, especially for the marginalised and excluded sections of society. Social capital is said to be built at different levels such as: Family, schools, local communities, firms, civil society, public sector, gender and ethnicity [OECD (2001), pp 45]. Not all forms of social capital are, however, good and some may lead to socially undesirable outcomes. The activities of terrorists, drug cartels etc fall under this category. Nevertheless, the benefits from most types overshadow the negative consequences [OECD (2001), pp 43].

Three basic forms namely (i) bonding (ii) bridging and (iii) linking social capital have so far been identified [Woolcock (1999)]. Bonding social capital refers to relations among family members and ethnic groups [OECD (2001), pp. 42] and this provides for denser networks [Sobel (2002), pp. 151]. Bridging social capital refers to relations with friends, associates and colleagues [OECD (2001), pp. 42] which creates larger networks [Sobel (2002), pp. 151]. Linking social capital refers to relations between different social strata in a hierarchy where power, social status and wealth are accessed by different groups [OECD (2001), pp. 42]. Linking social capital relates to the capability of individuals as well as communities to extract benefits (such as resources, ideas, information etc) from formal institutions which are beyond the community radius [Woolcock (2001)]. The benefits of high levels of integration or strong intra-community ties depend on the extent of linkage [Woolcock (1998), pp 174]. In other words, over time, intensive intra-community integration must give way to extensive extra-community linkages [Ibid, pp 175]. Several studies have proved this [Ibid].

The Influence of Social Capital

A miscellany of economic and non-economic benefits results from social capital. There is a positive relationship between social capital (measured as social networks) and education, child welfare, crime, health, happiness and democratic governments [see OECD (2001) pp 52-55]. Knack (1999) found that "social capital reduces poverty rates and improves, or at a minimum do not worsen, income inequality" and that "improving governmental and civil social capital are not the only ways, or necessarily the best ways, of reducing poverty" [pp. 28]. The creation of relationships between civil servants and local associations in north-east Brazil led to better implementation and performance of a health programme. More families were served and infant mortality decreased [Freedheim (1988)].

Micro level studies are the best examples of social capital at work. Even the probing "Can We Trust Social Capital" [Sobel (2002)] admits that "the most compelling work on social capital studies small group interactions" (pp. 151). Several such studies [D'Silva and Pai (2003), Chopra (2002), Mohapatra (2001), Mukherjee (2002), Krishna and Uphoff (1999) etc] draw our attention to the following key issues: (i) the role of trust, connectedness, networking, norms, collective action, leadership and institutional efficiency, (ii) the importance of dense networking among agents in and across sectors, their continuity, under evolving norms and rules for sustainable development, and (iii) the importance of comprehending regional sentiments and the existing socio-economic structure prior to the execution of plans. Development policies viewing people as agents of change must create an environment which promotes/ generates trust, linkages and networking between: (i) people, (ii) people and institutions and (iii) between institutions themselves (i.e. both formal and informal institutions).

Gugerty, Kremer et al (1999) examined the impact of development funding on the production of social capital in western Kenya in 2 settings viz., women's community groups and community primary schools. They found that different types of funding had different types of effects on social capital. While one form of social capital (internal solidarity and strength) was strengthened by development funding, other forms, such as linkages and networking, either reduced or remained unaffected. The net effect, according to the authors, would depend on the nature and purpose of the organization and the context in which funding takes place [Ibid. pp 23].

The World Bank's Dutch-supported program "Learning and Research on Culture and Poverty" is based on the notion that for development processes to be effective in reducing poverty, an understanding of culture is necessary. The reasons cited for this are: (i) culture influences what is valued in society and therefore shapes the ends of development that are valuable to the poor and, (ii) culture influences how individuals, communities, informal and formal institutions respond to developmental changes. Knowledge of culture(s) is a means to effective poverty reduction [http://www.worldbank.org/poverty/scapital/].

Implications for Policy Initiatives and Interventions

The UNDP's Human Development Report (HDR), 2004, like its earlier editions looks at development from a human development perspective. Human development, as it is perceived today, should allow people to live and lead the kind of life they wish to. But the kind of life that people want to lead and live are determined and fashioned by numerous factors which change over time as well. The variety of choices that can be made available depends upon the availability of funds and their efficient utilisation on targeted groups. The HDR (2004) report recognises and emphasises the effective management of cultural identities in multicultural societies for successful development outcomes. It goes on to say that human development goes beyond health, education, a decent living standard and political freedom and adds that expanding social, political and economic opportunities, do not automatically guarantee cultural freedom [pp 6]. Culture, of course, is an important source in the formation of human and social capital but whether management of cultural liberty is possible in multi ethnic societies (in terms of the costs involved) remains an open question. Most countries are culturally diverse and as per world population data of 2003, thirty (30) countries have less than 10 per cent of the world's ethnic or religious groups; 42 countries have between 10 – 25 per cent and 110 countries have more than 25 per cent ethnic or religious groups. A glance across the bottom 35 countries of the same index reveals that 30 are African countries. In these nations identities have been torn apart by the geographical and territorial demarcations executed by their colonial powers and bears resemblance to the North-Eastern States of India facing comparable predicaments. These poor countries and States, if one were to follow the Report's recommendations, are called upon to invest across their political boundaries to promote and manage cultural identity and liberty. Moreover their effective management (where the State has a major role to play and not simply maintain a status quo) entails the devolution of powers and the creation of more political spaces. In the absence of such management, further ethnic fragmentation and perusal of parochial interests will hinder the growth process. Reilly and Phillpot (2002) in a study of 19 provinces of Papua New Guinea with high degrees of autonomy and variations in economic performance found that government strength alone could not account for economic differences. Of the 5 indicators used, they found 3 measures viz. quality of education, level of community knowledge of current affairs and the number of women in local politics, to have significant correlation between social capital and economic development. On the other hand, using the number of community based organizations, as an indicator, in each province, demonstrated negative correlation with development. Hence, ethnic fragmentation can lead to lower levels of development by impeding social capital.

Heller (1996) made known that Kerela, through the politics of compromise and synergy, between a proactive State and a vibrant civil society, made great progress especially in terms of Human Development Index or HDI (despite its low per capita income). Though indicative of an equitable distribution of the growth proceeds, Kerela ranked low as per the HPI (Human Poverty Index). However, Kerela also had the highest incidence of unemployment at 8 million [NHDR (2001), pp 37]. Sufficient employment opportunities did not keep pace with its development status and this consequently led to massive migration of its population. The performances of some other Indian States are difficult to understand. For instance, Manipur ranks high in terms of both HDI and HPI, but one fails to understand as to how the decades of ethnic tensions and violence (persisting even today) has not negatively affected its HDI rank.

The above contradictions have important implications for policy and developmental interventions. Foremost, interventions must be context specific evolving with the needs of the time. Replication of successful models cannot provide the solution as generalised solutions do not exist. The brief literature review establishes that social cohesion is crucial for sustaining development and ushering economic prosperity in societies and such public policies ought to be pursued that facilitate the process of networking and strengthening social capital. But social interactions require a deeper understanding of where social capital comes from [Sobel (2002), pp 142] and sufficient time must be invested to comprehending the roots. But for a start, efficient implementation and enforcement of laws can instil trust thereby escalating networking (connectedness/ linkages). The factors promoting trust vary across regions and one must be sensitive to the heterogeneity. Where collective action problems arise, they can be overcome by balancing the conflicting interests, by self enforcing the norms/ rules of behaviour that involves a process of mutual monitoring [Ostrum, (1990)]. Local institutions can play a pivotal role in promoting inter and intra -group interactions.

People need to believe that they are a part of any process to develop a sense of ownership and responsibility. Sensitising of issues can ensure improved civic participation in the decision making process thereby shaping the quality of governance. Superior governance and proficient institutions go hand in hand in creating an enabling environment assisting the build up of human capabilities (by targeting the marginalised, poor, disadvantaged and the excluded sections).

A strong state, a vibrant civil society, and the nature of their interrelationship can determine the prospects of economic groups and their efficacy in shaping the willingness and ability of the state to act in a developmental manner [Woolcock (1998), pp 176]. A range of developmental outcomes is possible hinging on the "State's organisational capacity, and its engagement with and responsiveness to civil society" and this mandates a "more sophisticated understanding of the role of state-society relations in development [Ibid]. The effectiveness of a top-down or a bottom-up approach or a combination of both will largely depend on the resolving of the dilemmas associated with them [Ibid, pp 179]. For sustained economic development a dynamic interaction is necessary between the two. For the top-down approach "combinations of state-society relations (synergy) must coexist with cohesive corporate ties (integrity)" [Ibid, pp 180] while at the same time, for the bottom-up approach, "intensive extra-community ties (integration) must begin to coexist with more extensive albeit "weaker" extra-community networks (linkage)" [Ibid].

Conclusion

Development of human resource is a requisite for economic growth and development though the identification all factors affecting it, isn't an easy task. Outcomes (favourable or unfavourable) are the result of a complex set of interactions which change over time. But these outcomes/ indicators along with and a simplistic understanding of the interactions amplify the role of human and social capital in the process of development. Human capital and social capital are non- economic factors and multi-faceted. Subject to change, new forms constantly evolve to commensurate with the needs of time. Rapid technological changes in some sectors have necessitated higher skills and educational requirements.

Even though human and social capitals are not directly connected, they are mutually enforcing with positive externalities benefiting many people. Social capital is inherent in cultures and norms of behaviour, values and social organisations that change with time (new forms of social movements and civic participation). The growth /development process is complex one but in which, the organisation of society plays a significant role. In fact, the organisation of society at any point of time reflects "historical, cultural, social, political, and economic processes" [Greif cited in Woolcock (1998) pp 187]. An understanding of these factors can help find customised responses for specific groups.

Social capital helps to share information and overcome to some extent the market failures reflected by incomplete information. This can play an important role in poverty alleviation [Grootaert (1998), pp 4). The much written about success of the Grameen Bank of Bangladesh, a group- based lending scheme, is an illustration of the poorer have easier access to credit because the members had better information of each other. But the lack of economic opportunities may not raise incomes at the village level and thus, social capital needs to be combined with other forms of capital [Ibid, pp 6].

Social networking emerges as a key element is achieving socially desirable outcomes. Improved networking amid dissimilar economic agents personifies trust, and trust reduces costs and improves the efficiency and productivity of firms. Social and human capitals play significant roles in the development process and outcomes and therefore, even in the absence of ideal and comprehensive measures, their roles have become difficult to ignore.

REFERENCES

Coleman, J (1988): "Social Capital in the Creation of Human Capital". American Journal of Sociology, Vol. 94: Supplement, pp.s95-s120.

Collins, Randall (1994): *Four Sociological Traditions*, Oxford University Press, New York.

Chopra, Kanchan (2002): "Social Capital and Development Process: Role of Formal and Informal Institutions", Economic and Political Weekly (EPW), July 13, pp. 2911-2916.

D'silva, Emmanuel, And Sudha Pai (2003): "Social Capital and Collective Action: Development Outcomes in Forest Protection and Watershed Development", EPW, April 5, pp. 1404-1415.

Dreze, Jean and A. Sen (1998): *India: Economic Development and Social Opportunity*. Oxford University Press, Delhi.

Freedheim, S (1988): *Why Fewer Bells Toll in Ceara: Success of a Community Health Worker Program in Ceara, Brazil*, Master's Thesis, Massachusetts Institute of Technology, Cambridge, [in Groottaert (1998), pp 12].

Greif, Avner: "Cultural beliefs and the organisation of society," 944.

Groottaert, Christiaan (1998): "Social Capital: The Missing Link?" Social Capital Initiative, Working Paper No.3, World Bank.

Gugerty, M.K. and M. Kremer with S. Moulin, R. Namunyu and M. Wechuli (1999): Draft "The Impact of Development Funding on Social Capital: The Kenya Local Community Action Project",
[http://www.worldbank.org/poverty/scapital/]

Heller, P (1996): "Social Capital as a Product of Class Mobilization and State Intervention: Industrial Workers in Kerela, India". World Development, 24: pp. 1055-72.

Human Development Report (2004): "Cultural Liberty in Today's Diverse World", UNDP.

Kenkel, D. (1991): "Health Behaviour, Health Knowledge, and Schooling", *Journal of Political Economy*, Vol. 99, (2) pp. 287-305.

Knack, Stephen (1999): "Social Capital, Growth and Poverty: A Survey of Cross-Country Evidence", Social Capital Initiative; Working Paper No. 7, World Bank.

Krishna, Anirudh And Norman Uphoff (1999): "Mapping and Measuring Social Capital: A Conceptual and Empirical Study of Collective Action for Conserving and Developing Watersheds in Rajasthan, India", Social Capital Initiative, Working Paper no. 13, World Bank.

Krueger, A and Lindahl, M (1999): "Education for Growth in Sweden and the World", NBER Working Paper, No. 7190.

Mohapatra, Bishnu, N. (2001): "Social Connectedness and Fragility of Social Capital: View from an Orissa Village", EPW, February 24.

Mukherjee, Neela (2002): "Measuring Social Capital: Forest Committees in West Bengal", EPW, July 20, pp. 2994-2997.

National Human Development Report [NHRD], (2001), Planning Commission, Government of India, Oxford University Press, New Delhi.

OECD [Organisation For Economic Co-Operation And Development], (2001): *The Well-Being of Nations: The Role of Human and Social Capital*, OECD Publications, Paris.

Ostrom, Elinor (1990): *Governing the Commons: The Evolution of Institutions for Collective Action*, Cambridge, Cambridge University Press.

Raudenbush, S. W. and Kasim, R. M. (1998): "Cognitive Skills and Economic Inequality: Findings from the National Adult Literacy Survey", Harvard Educational Review, Vol. 68 (1) pp. 33 – 79.

Reilly, Benjamin And Robert Phillpot (2002): "Making Democracy Work in Papua New Guinea: Social Capital and Provincial Development in an Ethnically Fragmented Society", Asian Survey, Vol. 42, No. 6, pp. 906-27.

[http://www.worldbank.org/poverty/scapital/]

Sobel, Joel. (2002): "Can We Trust Social Capital?" Journal of Economic Literature, Vol. XL, pp 139-154.

Woocock, Michael (1998) "Social Capital and Economic Development: Toward a Theoretical Synthesis and Policy Framework", *Theory and Society* 27(2): pp. 151-208.

Woocock, Michael (1999): "Social Capital: The State of the Notion", Paper presented at a Multi –disciplinary Seminar on Social Capital: Global and Local Perspectives, Helsinki, April 15, [Cited in OECD (2001), pp. 42.]

Woocock, Michael (2001): "The Place of Social Capital in Understanding Social and Economic Outcomes", in J. F. Helliwell (ed.): *The Contribution of Human and Social Capital to Sustained Economic Growth: International Symposium Report*, Human Resources Development Canada and OECD, [Cited in OECD (2001): pp. 42.]

3

HUMAN DEVELOPMENT AND THE MANAGEMENT OF NATURAL RESOURCES: SOME BASIC ISSUES

– *Utpal Kumar De*

Introduction

Stock of natural resources and their utilization, to a large extent, determine the level and pace of development of a country. Though the development of technology and human resources can reduce the dependence on natural resources (both renewable and non-renewable), to a certain extent, there is a limit beyond which the substitution of natural resources is not possible. That is, even after accepting the Hartwick's (1977, 1995) weak sustainability criterion, we cannot deny the fact that a minimum stock of natural resources is always necessary for the continuous progress of an economy. All the resources are not unlimited in supply and not distributed uniformly across different regions and thus there is a need to exploit and utilize them judiciously. Otherwise, development process will not be sustainable as argued by the Club of Rome in *Limits to Growth* (Meadows et al, 1972). Judicious management is more crucial in case of exhaustible resources as these cannot be regenerated in a lifetime. Even in case of renewable natural resources, proper care and management is needed. These resources can also be vanished if their rate of exploitation is more than the rate of natural regeneration, i.e. due to over exploitation.

It is widely believed that open access exploitation of common property resources leads to rapid degradation and extinction of such resources (Hardin, G. 1968). So ownership pattern has some important bearing on the management of resources. But in some cases, mismanagement and overexploitation is also observed for resources under private ownership primarily due to lack of understanding, awareness, as well as knowledge. Incidence of poverty has also an important bearing on the degradation of natural resources especially the common resources.

Poverty and Natural Resource Interlinkage

Large number of poor people in the world live in remote areas and they are heavily dependent on the natural resources. Their level of income and quality of life are highly affected by the extent of environmental degradation. Also they are more vulnerable to the degraded environment and pollution than the richer people due to their nature of job. Therefore, with the rise in incidence of poverty, stress on environment and natural resource increase. As the poorer have less entitlement and access to education and health care facilities, their efficiency of work and income remain at low level. Also tendency of population growth among them is higher. So it leads to rise in pressure on environment and causes further degradation. The degraded environment again adversely affects their living conditions and thereby their quality of life. Hence it is essential to ensure sustainable environment for the survival of human being (World Bank, 1987, 1988).

Thus, there is a close association between level of human resource development and the management and quality of environment. If the level of human development is high, especially per capita income and education, management of natural resources will be better and degradation will be less and vice versa. On the other hand if per capita availability of natural resources is less, the development of human resources will be poor, which in turn leads to further degradation of natural resources.

The present chapter tries to explain the nexus between nature of human resource development and the management of natural resources or environmental quality with a special stress on North-East India, where the incidence of poverty is notable.

The plan of the chapter is as follows: In the next section, interlinkage among the different indicators of human resource development (HRD)is explained. It is followed by a brief discussion of how the quality of environmental resources affect and are being affected by human resource. Thereafter, the circular and multidimensional linkages among poverty, human capital and environment or natural resource is analysed with the help of some empirical facts and figures. Then the changes in dependence and stress on natural resources especially land and forest over time in North East India is reviewed. The relationship between changes in forest cover and variation in incidence of poverty and per capita income is examined with the help of data from North East Indian states. The final section includes the conclusion and policy implications emanated from the observations and overall discussion.

Indicators of HRD and Their Interlinkage

Level of human development depends on a number of variables like the level of income, nutritional intake, technology, level of education, health care and natural resources etc. There are three basic indicators of Human Resource Development (HRD). (a) Income indicator : Per Capita Gross Domestic Product that measures the standard of living of the people of a region; (b) life expectancy at birth : that is an index of the longevity of life or standard of attainment of health care and (c) index of educational achievement : calculated by the combination of adult literacy rate and gross enrolment ratio at all levels with weights 2/3 and 1/3. The three indicators that determine the level of human development are also closely interlinked as is shown in the Flow Chart 3.1.

Flow Chart-3.1

Interlinkage among the three indicators

Higher GDP per capita

↓

Better entitlement and access to education & health care facilities

↓

Increase efficiency and productivity of the people and help controlling propulation

↓

Growth of economy and rising GDP per head

At micro level, the cluster of factors like nutrition, health, formal education and training all are embodied in an individual and these factors provide the individual some advantage over the others without them.

A healthier, better-educated person is capable of producing more. Therefore the commitment of current resources or income to improving an individual's health and education leads to increase in that person's future productivity and income (Bardhan and Udry, 1999; P. 123). At macro level, a country with higher GDP per capita has better entitlement or affordability and possibility of better access to education and health care facilities. As the rich country can afford to acquire more of these goods, their capabilities of technological innovation, efficiency and thus productivity is higher. Moreover, having better understanding and knowledge, they can adopt better measures for population control. Ultimately it accelerates the growth of the economy and per capita GDP again.

Therefore it is natural that the developed industrialized countries have higher adult literacy and enrolments at all levels and thus acquire better knowledge and also have better health care facilities and hence higher life expectancy at birth. On the other hand, the low-income countries in general have low adult literacy (in most cases first generation is literate), though the enrolment ratio has been rising at the primary level (due to special public policies and efforts of different governments) dropout is increasing at higher order and access to health care is also poor and thus life expectancy at birth is less. Hence human resource development is poor.

Environment and HRD

Like income and human capital circular linkage, there exists a circular relationship between the natural resource and environmental quality and human resource development. The Flow Chart 3.2 reveals that scant availability of natural resources and poor environmental quality is associated with low productivity, output and income. This provides people with less scope to achieve standard education and health care facilities. Thus poor human resource development leads to further mismanagement and more rampant use and degradation of environmental quality and natural resources.

Data available on degradation of forest and human resource development at cross country level show that degradation of forest is very low in the countries that acquired very high human development (Human Development Report, 2000). Only in Bahamas average annual deforestation during 1990-95 was 2.6 per cent. In Japan, Finland, Korea, Brunei Darussalam, Argentina and Chile it was merely 0.1, 0.1, 0.2, 0.6, 0.3 and 0.4 per cent respectively. In other cases there was either no degradation or improvement in forest area. On the other hand, degradation of forest is comparatively higher in most of the countries that achieved medium or low level of human development (Human Development Report, 2000). It was 7.5, 8.1, 2.6, 3.5, 2.6, 2.5, 2.9, 2.4, 2.2, 3.1 and 5.8 percent in Jamaica, Lebanon, Paraguay, Philippines, Thailand, Jordan, Pakistan, Malaysia, Panama, Costa Rica and Comoros respectively.

Flow Chart-3.2

How Environment affect Human Resource Development ?

Natural resource and Environmental quality
↓
Productivity, output and income
↓
Access to education and health care
↓
Human resource development

Poverty, Human Capital and Natural Resource Use

People living below poverty line mostly belong to the remote areas and their living conditions are directly affected by the availability of critical natural resources in their surroundings. But the standard poverty measures do not include the value of those directly derived by the poor from the nature. So in many cases, the magnitude of poverty is overstated and therefore the actual effect of changes in natural resource availability on poverty is not focused properly.

In most cases, the poor earn their livelihood directly from the environment (e.g., from common forest they collect fuel wood, timber, leaves and herbs for building cottage, extract food articles and some other things to sell and earn. Also they use grazing field for raising livestock, harvest common fisheries, water bodies for drinking water and so on) (Jodha, 1986). Moreover, due to limited access to education, heath care and awareness, tendency of population growth is relatively higher among them, which put more pressure on environment and accelerate the process of environmental degradation and thereby reduce the productive capacity of those natural resources. This, in turn, affects their livelihood through declining impact on their income and material collected from the nature, which means lower human development.

Thus, when a country starts developing and per capita GDP grows, unless it is accompanied by reduction in inequality and the development in the field of healthcare, education and awareness among the people commensurate with the proper public policy (tax, subsidy, quota etc), environmental quality is bound to degrade.

One exception is that the poor are not always responsible for environmental degradation. In many cases due to the better accessibility and encouraging government policy (e.g., subsidies for fossil fuels or large scale commercial fishing fleets), the rich cause much more damage to the environment than the poor. They do the damage primarily due to their unsustainable luxurious consumption of natural resources, their profit oriented behaviour and they are responsible for the creation of large-scale industrial waste and pollution (without taking proper measure for treatment), the burden of which has been mostly shouldered by the vulnerable poor.

On the other hand, many of the poor do not have proper access to those resources (may be due to lack of property right or capabilities) and even in some cases they are found to invest and judiciously manage (due to their indigenous knowledge) of those. Whatever damage they do is mainly for their survival. Their income, opportunities and health are highly affected by the depletion or degradation of natural resources.

(1) Around 900 million poor people are living in rural areas in the world and depend on natural products for much of their livelihoods. Most of their diseases occur due to environmental risk factors.

(2) Almost half the world's poorest people, i.e., more than 500 million (by the most conservative estimates) live on

marginal land. Under current policies and conditions, the number is expected to rise to 800 million by 2020. The livelihood of these people is directly and acutely affected by natural resource degradation.

(3) More than 1.5 billion people live in dry-lands, which is almost 35 per cent of developing world's population — about 37 per cent of the people in Asia (1.1 billion) and 34 per cent in Sub-Saharan Africa (180 million), 59 per cent in the Arab States (140 million) and 26 per cent in Latin America and the Caribbean (120 million) (Human Development Report, 1997).

(4) Soil degradation alone each year (due to improper use and maintenance of land) affects nearly two billion hectares, damaging the livelihood of around one billion people living on dry lands.

(6) Around 70 per cents of commercial fisheries in the world are fully or over-exploited.

(7) One-third of the developing world's population are facing safe drinking water crisis and the same will go on increasing unless proper measures are undertaken (Human Development Report, 1997).

Sustainable management of environment is thus an important requirement so that the ecosystem can provide services to sustain human livelihood and support for the improvement of the components of human development. Hence withering poverty, inequality and ensuring food security, environmental sustainability is among the major UN Millennium Development Goals declared in 2000.

Flow Chart 3.3 shows the downward spiral movement of poverty, human capital and environmental quality/natural resource. The vicious circle of poverty and environment will continue if there is poverty, low educational and health care achievement and degraded environment in the beginning. Thus there will be continuous mounting of pressure on natural resource and decline in their availability unless the linkage is broken either through proper environment care, sustainable resource management and striking against poverty simultaneously.

Flow Chart-3.3

How Poverty & HD is linked with Environment ?

Incidence of Poverty
- → Low educational and health care facilities
  - → Higher population growth
    - → Pressure on Natural resource and Environment & Poor Management
      - → Degradation of environment
        - → Low productivity and income
          - → Incidence of Chronic poverty

Further Environmental Degradation

Stress on Natural Resource in North East India

The economies of all the states of North East India (NEI) are primarily agricultural. Though there has been decline in dependence on primary activities, still now majority of the people are engaged in primary sector. This is clear from Table-3.1 that shows the changes in sector-wise distribution of main workers during 1971 to 1991. The reduction in dependence on agriculture has been very slow across all the North Eastern states. However, the supply of primary input of agriculture i.e., land is fixed. But population continued to grow at rapid rates in all these states. Thus per capita availability of usable land has been decreasing as is shown in Table-3.2. As majority of people are still engaged in agriculture and allied activities, pressure on land has been increasing. Also, fallow period of shifting cultivation has been falling drastically (from 17 - 20 years in 1970s to 2 - 3 years). Further the methods adopted to increase the productivity of land in many cases leads to decline in long run productivity of soil. Moreover conversion of forestland has been taking place to make up the shortage of cultivable land and to meet the need of increased population. So degradation of forest has been taking place to meet the increasing need of the people. The method of shifting cultivation that is widely practised in North East India is also partly responsible for the degradation of forest (Reddy et al., 2001).

Table-3.1
Changes in the Sector-wise Distribution of Main Workers in North East India from 1971 to 1991

	% of Main Workers in Primary Sector		% of Main Workers in Secondary Sector		% of Main Workers in Tertiary Sector	
State	1971	1991	1971	1991	1971	1991
Arunachal	80.44	67.44	0.45	8.66	19.11	23.96
Assam	77.04	73.99	4.20	5.56	17.86	20.45
Manipur	71.30	70.00	12.24	9.66	16.46	20.34
Meghalaya	81.84	74.81	3.30	3.74	14.86	21.46
Mizoram	84.17	65.99	1.76	5.07	14.07	28.94
Nagaland	79.46	75.26	2.38	3.48	18.16	21.26
Tripura	76.58	64.08	4.25	6.41	19.17	29.51
N-E India	77.45	72.61	4.93	5.78	17.62	21.61
All India	72.56	67.50	10.69	12.00	16.75	20.50

Source: (1) Basic Statistics of North Eastern Region, 2002 (2) NEDFi, Report, 2002

Table-3.2
Per-Capita Availability of Land in North East India (Hectare)

State	1971	1981	1991	2001
Arunachal	12.07	8.86	6.36	5.04
Assam	0.54	0.39	0.35	0.29
Manipur	2.06	1.56	1.20	0.93
Meghalaya	2.22	1.68	1.26	0.97
Mizoram	6.52	4.26	3.03	2.35
Nagaland	3.20	1.79	1.28	0.79
Tripura	0.67	0.5	0.38	0.33
N-E India	1.16	0.84	0.71	0.58
All India	0.55	-	0.36	0.30

Source: (1) Basic Statistics of North Eastern Region, 2002
(2) NEDFi, Report, 2002.

Poverty, Per-Capita Income and Forest Cover in NEI

Incidence of poverty coupled with rapid population growth, which is also due to low human capital formation, lead to decline in per capita availability of forest resources and accelerate forest degradation (Rao, 1994; De, 2003). Though there has been decline in incidence of poverty across all North Eastern states, it is still higher than the national average. The rate of decline also varies across the states. The highest rate of decline was observed in the state of Mizoram (from 36 per cent in 1983 to only 19.47 per cent in 1999-2000) i.e., by 45.92 per cent where literacy and other human development indices are also higher. It was lowest in Assam where percentage of poverty declines from 40.47 in 1983 to 36.09 in 1999-2000 i.e., by only 10.82 per cent. Table-3.3 shows the rate of change in incidence of poverty in North Eastern states during 1983 to 2000.

Table-3.3

Changes in poverty in North East India (Percentage)

	Incidence in Percentage			Changes in Percentage		
State	1983	1993-94	1999-00	1983 to 1993-4	1993-4 to 1999-00	1983 to 1999-00
Arunachal	40.38	39.35	33.47	-2.55	-14.94	-17.11
Assam	40.47	40.86	36.09	0.96	-11.67	-10.82
Manipur	37.02	33.78	28.54	-8.75	-15.51	-22.91
Meghalaya	38.81	37.92	33.87	-2.29	-10.68	-12.73
Mizoram	36.00	25.66	19.47	-28.72	-24.12	-45.92
Nagaland	39.25	37.92	32.67	-3.39	-13.84	-16.76
Tripura	40.03	39.01	34.44	-2.55	-11.71	-13.96

Source: Planning Commission.

The theory of Environmental Kuznets Curve (EKC) says that the degradation of environment first rises with the rise in per capita income and reaches a maximum and thereafter it declines with further rise in per capita income due to positive income elasticity of demand for environmental quality (Shafik and Bandyopadhyay, 1992; Seldon and Song, 1994; Grossman and Krueger, 1995). Therefore a similar kind of relationship is expected to exit due to the same cause between quality of environment/ natural resource and different components of human resource development like per capita GDP, educational achievement and longevity of life. Spread of education makes people more conscious about the management of natural resources. Moreover rise in income helps people accessing more health care and hence raises life expectancy at birth. On the other hand, management of resources is essential for maintaining the productivity and earning of the people. As forest is one of the major natural resource of North East India and mostly are open access common forest even if owned by the community or the government, we tried to look into the relationship between degradation of forest and Per Capita Income as well as incidence of poverty. It may be expected that in the initial phase when per capita income is very less but growing that will be associated with the rising stress on forest and thus more degradation. Where as when per capita income rises and alternative opportunities and the substitutes come up, damage of forest will be reduced and hence rising per capita income will be associated with the better availability of forest resources in the later stage. Taking the cross-state figures of poverty, changes in poverty, per capita income and calculating their correlation with the changes in forest cover across the North eastern states we tried to arrive at the results in which the solution to the problem of forest degradation will be lying (Table- 3.4).

Table-3.4
Poverty, Per-Capita Income and Changes in Forest Cover in North East India

State	Poverty in 1999-2000, Percentage	Per Capita Income 1999-2000 (at 1993-94 prices)	Changes in Forest Cover in 1995-97 (Sq. Km)	Changes in Percentage	
				1993-94 to 1999-00	1983 to 1999-00
(1)	(2)	(3)	(4)	(5)	(6)
Arunachal	33.47	9170	-19	-14.94	-17.11
Assam	36.09	5978	-94	-11.67	-10.82
Manipur	28.54	7231	-140	-15.51	-22.91
Meghalaya	33.87	7826	-55	-10.68	-12.73
Mizoram	19.47	8109	199	-24.12	-45.92
Nagaland	32.67	9118*	-70	-13.84	-16.76
Tripura	34.44	6813	4	-11.71	-13.96

R_{24} = -0.723, R_{34} =, R_{45} = -0.77, R_{46} = -0. 792, R_{43} = 0.233

Note: (1) * For Nagaland the data on per capita income was taken from 1998-99 year as it was not available for 1999-00.

(2) R_{ij} represents the correlation between i^{th} and j^{th} column.

Concluding Remarks

From the correlation results we observe that there is a significantly inverse correlation between the incidence of poverty and the degradation of forest. Also we observe similar kind of inverse relationship between the changes in poverty and the degradation of forest. The results indicate that the degradation of forest (either due to shifting cultivation or other reasons) increases with the decline in poverty in North East India.

Similarly we observe that the correlation between changes in forest cover and per capita income is positive but not so strong. It indicates that as per capita income rises, even if we take the annual compound rate of degradation of forest during 1989 to 1999, a similar result is observed.

The results may appear to be inconsistent. The fact is that all the North Eastern states have per capita income well below the national average. Moreover it is associated with high inequality, which is clear from the incidence of poverty. Hence many of the families still face the survival problem and hence they earn mostly from the forest. Poor do survive at the expense of easily accessible forest resource.

The positive correlation between per capita income and degradation of forest is due to fact that theses states are still in rising phase of Environmental Kuznets Curve (EKC). Per capita income of all these states is well below the national average (over Rs 10000) per capita income. They are yet to reach the peak per capita income and the technology after which their dependence on forest will be declining and they will have the alternative opportunities. But the positive relationship between per capita income and degradation of forest is not significant, which may be because of the government policies and initiatives through joint forest management, community forestry, social forestry programmes etc that help protecting and regenerating many forest areas during last two decades. Andrew Foster has shown that economic development in India was associated with the rise in demand for natural resource (forest resource) which led to an increase in its supply during 1971 to 1999 (Smith, 2003). Among these states, Mizoram and Tripura occupy top two positions in terms of educational achievement (e.g., higher literacy rate and enrolment ratio) and we observe improvement in forest resource in them.

Promoting environmental sustainability through participatory management of natural resources by involving local people remains an option for the continuous improvement of standard of living and thus human capital in the long run. It would also help proper monitoring and protecting the environmental standard. For this property right (De, 2003) of the stakeholders should be clearly defined to avoid any kind of conflict and adverse effect.

Secondly, proper government policy (pricing of resources, tax-subsidies etc) is needed for the conservation and maintaining its service to the people. Merely legislation will not be sufficient.

Thirdly, strong actions are needed to strike and eradicate extreme poverty.

Fourthly, investment in science and technology for the generation of alternative source of energy and opportunities to reduce the stress on environment is the need of the hour. Lastly, spread of education especially environmental education may raise awareness and understanding among the people so that they can manage resources judiciously.

In conclusion we can say that, sustainable environmental management, poverty eradication, spread of universal education, reduction of child mortality through better health care need to be addressed simultaneously. Without good environment other targets cannot be achieved. Also without better education and removal of hunger, better environment cannot be ensured.

REFERENCES

Bardhan P. and C. Udry, (1999), *Development Microeconomics*, Oxford University Press, New York.

De, U. K. (2003), "Economic Incentive and Environmental Management: A Study of Forestry in North East India", in Z. Husain (ed.) *Environmental Issues of North East India*, Regency Publications, New Delhi, pp. 170-188.

Grossman and Krueger (1995), "Economic Growth and the Environment", *The Quarterly Journal of Economics*, May, pp. 353-377.

Hardin, G. (1968), "The Tragedy of the Commons", *Science*, Vol. 162, pp. 1243-1247.

Hartwick, J. M. (1977) "Intergenerational Equity and the Investing of rent from Exhaustible Resources", *American Economic Review,* vol. 67. pp. 972 – 974.

Hartwick, J. M. (1995), "Sustainability and Consumption Path in Open Economies with Exhaustible Resources", *Review of International Economics,* Vol. 3, pp. 275-283.

Jodha, N. S. (1986), "Common Property Resources and Rural Poor in Dry Regions of India", *Economic and Political Weekly,* Vol. 21, No. 27, pp. 1169-1181.

Meadows, D. H., et al. (1972), *The limits to Growth,* Universe Books, New York.

North Eastern Council, Government of India, *Basic Statistics of North Eastern Region,* Various Issues.

Rao, C. H. H. (1994), *Agricultural Growth, Rural Poverty and Environmental Degradation in India,* Oxford University Press, New Delhi, pp. 88-89.

Ratna Reddy, V., et.al. (2001), "Forest Degradation in India: Extent and Determinants", *Indian Journal of Agricultural Economics,* Vol. 56, No. 4, pp. 631-651.

Seldon and Song (1994), "Environmental Quality and Development: Is There a Kuznets Curve for Air Pollution Emissions?" *Journal of Environmental Economics and Management,* Vol. 27, pp. 147-162.

Smith, J. M. (2003), *Wood Demand may lead to Forest Growth,* downloaded from the website http://espn.go.com/outdoors/conservation/news/2003/0812/1594600.html

Shafik, N. and S. Bandyopadhyay (1992), "Economic Growth and Environmental Quality: Time Series and Cross Section Evidence", World Bank Policy Research Working Paper// WPS904, Washington, D. C.: The World Bank.

World Bank (1987), *Environmental Growth and Development,* Development Committee Pamphlet 14, World Bank, Washington D. C.

World Bank (1988), *Environment and Development: Implementing the World Bank's New Policies,* Development Committee Pamphlet 17, World Bank, Washington D. C.

World Bank (1995, 1997, 2005), *Human Development Report.*

4

HUMAN DEVELOPMENT AND INHUMAN GROWTH

– *Gorky Chakraborty*

Introduction

Various changes during recent past have few parallels in human history. The world has progressed in many unique ways and directions which are reflected in technological, economic and industrial developments. In the process, there has also been enhancement in human capabilities, facilities and quality of life. But behind this veil of remarkable progress, the irony lies that the fruits of development have eluded the growing numbers of poor around the world. This has raised doubts regarding the 'form', 'content' and 'reach' of the development model being pursued currently. It has also raised serious issues concerning the choice between people's welfare vis-a-vis corporate profits. The certain lack of 'humane content' in our development model, whereby a 'selected few' flourishes and 'silent majority' perishes can neither be sustainable nor humane. Hence the search for an alternative development paradigm. The quest for human development through the betterment of various human development indices has been a small but significant step in that direction.

Mankind's concern for human development is age old. Aristotle's caution that 'wealth is evidently not the good we are seeking; for it is merely useful and for the sake of something else' is an insight in that direction (Ross : 1980). Marx while warning against 'commodity fetishism' argued for a reorientation of economic preoccupations. In his words, it will be seen how in place of the wealth and poverty of political economy come the rich human being and rich human need. The rich human being is simultaneously in need of a totality of human life activities (Marx : 1844)'. Amartya Sen in recent times have shown empirically that 'until a person or a group is endowed with capabilities, s/he or they will not be in a position to exchange their entitlements for sustaining livelihoods no matter what the levels of economic growth are (Dreze and Sen : 1989). Haq on the other states, 'the ultimate end of all development strategies must be people and their welfare : economic growth is only a means. Income generation is necessary, but it is not sum total of human life' (Haq : 1994) Thus in all the above expositions, development of human-being or human development takes the centre-stage where economic growth is a means to achieve the development goal.

Human Development and South Asia[1]

A comparison of income level and human development level is revealing. It shows the extent to which income and economic growth have been actually translated into human lives. For instance, Saudi Arabia has 15 times the per capita income of Jamaica, but 4 times its child mortality. United States ranks 6th in the world according to its per capita income, but 44th according to its child mortality rate. Similarly there are variations both within a nation and a region; within rural and urban areas; within gender, religion and ethnic groups. Therefore utmost caution should be exercised while generalizing human development indices over a large area or population groups, e.g. South Asia. But certain broad conclusions can certainly be inferred upon—

- three-quarters of the world illiterates live in five most populous Asian countries-China, India, Pakistan, Bangladesh and Indonesia;

- over 700 million people in Asia are in absolute poverty, over 600 million people who cannot read or write, two-thirds of them are women. Moreover about half of the population in the region have no access to safe drinking water ;
- the share of South Asia in global income is 2 percent but its share in global arms import is 20 per cent. Many countries in the region spend several times more on their military than on education and health. Soldiers out number teachers in many of them : Afghanistan and Laos have twice as many soldiers than teachers. Vietnam has three times as many;
- on the expenditure side, annual per capita expenditure on human priority areas are extremely low in South Asia : $2 in Bangladesh, $3 in Pakistan and Indonesia, $9 in India;
- on the other hand despite the persistence of grinding poverty, Asia receives a per capita ODA (Overseas Development Assistance) of only $4 compared to $26 for Africa, $16 for Middle East and $10 for Latin America;
- presently developing countries suffer a potential annual loss of atleast $50 billion from textile protectionism, $100 billion from agricultural subsidies in the industrial countries and another $100 billion from restrictions in trade-in-services. In other words, a market loss five times as large as the total foreign assistance they receive every year (HDR : 2004).

In the light of the figures mentioned above, the state of human development in South Asia can be easily understood. Although some of the nations in this region has experienced higher arithmetical growth figures, that have not yet translated into overall human development. This has, in turn, transformed the region into a hot-bed of various disturbing trends ranging from war, man-made natural disasters, insurgencies and increasing tide of fundamentalist outcries.

Human Development and India

It has been more than five decades since we embarked upon our 'tryst with destiny' to end poverty, hunger and unemployment. India seems to be at a vital crossroads today. On one hand we have the Indian 'rich' whose asset, income and lifestyles are easily comparable with their counterparts in various global metropolis, while on the other, more than one-third of the world's absolute poor reside in India. More than 75 million children are not in school and 216 million people without access to safe drinking water. Our development model, which in more than one way is an extension of the current global development trend has therefore several question marks. And thus the need to ascertain where do we stand in terms of human development indicators.

India has been sliding down the human development ladder and its fall has been much steeper during recent years. During 1991, India's HDI ranking has been 123rd which went down to 127th during 2004. This in itself speaks volumes about the state of affairs in India.

In terms of $1 criteria, absolute poor constitutes 34.7 percent of India's total population. In terms of average per capita income, the world figure is $5860 and for developing nations has been $1860 but for India it is way below at $460. So even during the years of so-called higher rates of economic growth in terms of per capita income, India has been way behind the level of developing nations.

The gender scenario in India shows signs of imminent concern. India lags far behind the world female literacy rate. It is 71.48 percent for the world as a whole whereas in India it is just 54.16 percent. India also has the dubious distinction of having the highest number of female death during childbirth. Even in terms of sex ratio there has been a sharp decline from 945 females per 1000 male to 927 during 1990-91 to 2001. This is certainly a disturbing trend, which seems to be more acute among developed and prosperous regions in India.

In global terms, on an average a man works for 403 minutes and a woman works for 423 minutes per day. But this gap is huge in India. Men work for 391 minutes while women work for 457 minutes. In contrast women in India earn 37.7 percent less than their male counterparts.

Even though there has been a recent surge in literacy rates in India yet it is far behind the average of developing nations, leave aside the developed states. Literacy among its citizens who are above 15 years of age is 61.3 percent while for developing nations it stands at 76.7 percent. The picture is bleaker in terms of infant and child mortality rates. Infant mortality is 56 per thousand live births worldwide whereas it is 67 for India. For child mortality the rates are 81 and 93 respectively.

One can go on quoting innumerable statistics highlighting the lower standards of human development in India. The need however, is for a reorientation of our development model whereby more emphasis is laid to tackle the human development problems instead of bothering ourselves solely with GNP figures.

Human Development and NER[2]

The North Eastern Region (NER) comprising of seven states of the Indian Union - Arunachal Pradesh, Assam, Manipur, Meghalaya, Mizoram, Nagaland and Tripura has a combined population of 38.5 million representing 3.8 percent of India's population and geographically cover 8.05 percent of the country's total area. Economically, these states are behind the national average and regarded as special category states. In terms of human development, the region presents us with a mixed picture.

States like Mizoram, Nagaland, Tripura, Manipur and Assam have overall literacy rates which are higher than national average. Except Arunachal Pradesh, all other states in the region have higher female literacy rates than their Indian counterparts.

Similarly the urban literacy rates of all the states are higher than the national average. All the states have a gross enrolment rate at primary level exceeding 90 percent. But there are gender disparities regarding enrolment among the states of the region. Except for Meghalaya, enrolments of girls are lower than boys. Similarly, except for Arunachal Pradesh, urban enrolment rates are lower than the rural enrolment rates in the region.

The higher enrolment rates in the NER are undoubtedly a positive sign but the inability to retain the students in the school is a big drawback which leads to dropouts. Rural areas have a higher dropout rates than urban areas and in some states the figures are absolutely shocking e.g. 80.99 percent in Meghalaya, 7 percent in Nagaland and 70.67 percent in Arunachal Pradesh. In urban areas, Arunachal Pradesh has the highest dropout rate at 58.71 percent, which is equally higher for boys (61.08 percent) and girls (55.72 percent). Other than Assam and Manipur, in all other states dropouts of girls are lower than that of boys at the primary level.

Mizoram and Nagaland have made good progress in opening up neighbourhood schools. But in Arunachal Pradesh and Meghalaya more than 50 percent of the villages have their schools located at a distance of more than the 2 kms. norms. Mean year of schooling is highest in Manipur (3.43 years) and lowest in Meghalaya (1.81 years). In all the above mentioned aspects of enrolment, drop outs and mean years of schooling, gender disparities within the region are far less than compared to other states in India.

The number of hospital beds available per 1000 population is a good indicator of health infrastructure. At the national level, 0.73 beds are available for 1000 population. In NER, Mizoram (1.67), Arunachal Pradesh (1.27), Meghalaya (0.99), Nagaland (0.91) and Manipur (0.79) the availability is higher than the national average. Assam (0.06) and Tripura (0.55) lag way behind in terms of this indicator.

Average life expectancy, although a good health indicator for the population, is difficult to assess for the region due to unavailability of related data. In Assam (the only state where data are available) expectation of life at birth for male is 58.7 years whereas for female it is 58.5 years, which are much lower compared to 60.6 and 61.7 years at the national level. Moreover women in Assam are certainly worse off in terms of health, wholesome food and nutrition due to which their average life expectancy is lower than male, an imminent sign of concern when compared with the all India pehnomenon.

Total dependency ratio in NER is highest in Meghalaya (892) followed by Assam (842) and Tripura (831). Rural dependency is highest in Meghalaya (947) while urban dependency is highest in Mizoram (710). In all cases young dependent ratio is far greater than old dependent ratio.

Mean age at marriage for female are highet in Mizoram 20.3 years and lowest in Tripura at 17.8 years. In rural areas it is highest in Nagaland 20.3 years and in urban areas it is highest in Mizoram at 20.7 years. Tripura has the lowest mean age at marriage for both urban and rural areas. Higher literacy levels in Mizoram may have played an important role in raising the mean age of marriage for their female citizens.

Infant and child mortality rates in NER portray a mixed picture. Infant mortality is highest in Assam (92) followed by Arunachal Pradesh (91), Tripura (82) and Meghalaya (80). Manipur (28) has the lowest rate while Nagaland (51) and Mizoram (58) are way above. Child mortality is highest in Arunachal Pradesh (139) followed by Assam and Tripura (101). As per the gender divide, infant mortality among girls are higher in Meghalaya, Mizoram, Nagaland and Tripura whereas girls outnumbers boys in case of child mortality in Manipur and Nagaland.

Monthly per capita consumption expenditure is a good economic indicator, which throws sufficient light on poverty and quality of life. Nagaland has the highest MPCE at Rs. 367 while it is lowest in Assam at Rs. 169.93. In rural areas Mizoram has the highest at Rs. 245.40 while Assam has the lowest at Rs. 153.60. It clearly highlights the levels of poverty in Assam compared to other states in NER. This is also highlighted in the per capita income figures of Assam within the region.

Conclusion

'Ever wondered what one human life is worth ? One person in a country like the United States is worth 1.5 million dollars, while a person in Russia is worth 300,000 dollars, a person in India or Tunisia worth 150,000 dollars' (Sinha: 1995). How can human lives have such price differentials ? In a world where a handful of economist from the developed countries are busy in preparing these inhuman statistics, the question arises whether our development model will solely be ruled by GNP figures or will we assign due weightage to the human indicators ? To any concerned person, GNP growth is a means towards human development and not an end in itself. The question that one confronts is how far have we been successful in implementing these goals into reality ? Are we blindfolded by the slogan that GNP growth rates are the only indicator of development ? Do the process of liberalization for global finance capital and its ever-increasing appetite for speculative profits, the only indicator of development ? Or, are there certain inherent contradictions within our development model, which does not allow us to implement a participatory human development programme ? An insight in resolving these contradictions is certainly necessary.

Markets may be impressive economically or technically. But they are of little value if they do not serve human development. Markets are the means, human development is the end. This has been true earlier and is equally true in today's era of finance-capital led globlization. For a country like India, which has extremely low levels of human development, the state should reorient itself towards peoples welfare instead of projecting itself as the sole *messiah* of supervising corporate profits. The Indian economy allegedly had a higher growth rate during 90's yet the rising number of poor, undernourished and unemployed has become a matter of serious concern during the same period. In other words has a higher arithmetic figure of economic growth rate transformed India into a 'republic of hunger'? If so, then should this be regarded as development ?

Scenario in NER is so different from the Indian milieu although the region represents certain healthy trends particularly in enrolment of students at primary level along with lesser gender disparities. A major area of focus in the region should be upon creating sustainable socio-economic inrastructures in rural areas. Without which all the states in the region will have higher dropout rates, higher illiteracy, lower health standards, higher infant and child mortality and lower life expectancy. But while trying to achieve these desired goals, the traditional wisdom, the participatory tribal ethos and historical patterns of occupational specialization should be taken into consideration. Moreover India's north-east should never be considered in an a historical fashion and neither its uniqueness be confused with exclusivism.

About twenty districts of the region have been identified as backwards in terms of several human development indicators.[3] Policy framers should prepare perspective plans for each of these districts after understanding the causes of human deprivation and therefore highlighting areas of concern. Community participation along with government and non-government delivery mechanism should be devised so that the 'people' for whom the plans are framed and implemented derive sustainable benefits. After all human development is not only limited to the creation of human capabilities but also how these capabilities are used productively and creatively for the betterment of humanity.

NOTES

1. All the figures quoted in this section are referred from (Haq : 1994)
2. All the **figures** quoted in this section are referred from *East India Human Development Report, 2004* (New Delhi : Oxford University Press, 2004).
3. Districts namely, Tawang, East Kameng, Jaintia Hills, South Garo Hills, West Garo Hills in Meghalaya; and Barpeta, Goalpara, Darrang, Bongaingaon, Sonitpur, Morgaon and Karbi Anglong in Assam have lower human development indicators compared to both within the respective states and the north eastern region as a whole. Indicators concerning literacy, female literacy, infant and child mortality, mean age of marriage of married female etc. bears testimony to lower human development levels among the above-mentioned districts.

REFERENCES

Dreze, Jean and Sen, Amartya, *Hunger and Public Action* (New Delhi : Oxford University Press, 1989).

Haq, Mahbul Ul, 'Human Development in India' in *Selected Readings* (Mussoorie: Lal Bahadur Shastri National Academy of Administration, 1994).

Human Development Report, 2004 (New Delhi : Oxford University Press, 2004).

Marx, Karl, *The Economic and Philsophic Manuscript of 1844* (London : Lawrence and Wishart, 1844).

Mahbub Ul Haq as quoted by Chetia, Dibyananda, *'Human development Among Tea Garden Labourers of Assam - A Case Study,'* an unpublished Ph. D. Thesis, Dibrugarh University, 2003.

Ross, D. (ed.) *Aristotle : The Nimochean Ethics* (Oxford University Press, 1980).

Wysham, Daphne, 'Ever Wondered What One Human Life is Worth ?' as quoted by Sinha, Amarjeet, 'Towards Evolution of a Concrete Agenda for Sustainable Development in India', *The Administrator,* Vol. XI, No. 2, April-June 1995.

Section - II
Education, Income and Human Development

5

HUMAN RESOURCE AND ITS STATUS IN NORTH-EAST INDIA

– Keya Sengupta

Introduction

Although the north eastern region of India has achieved some extent of economic development over the last few decades, yet the region is still a low income region, with a large number of its population in absolute poverty. This is, inspite of the existence of huge amount of natural resources. The prosperity of the entire region therefore depends on the effective use of its human resources, which can gear the economy of the region into the right channels for rapid economic development. Development of all developed nations and the success of economic reform in South East Asian nations has largely been shaped by their human resource. In the opposite case, inadequate development of human resources in the less developed nations, has lead to massive under development as the human engine of growth has not been able to channelise the economy into the right path of development. After all, it is the adequate development of human resources, which increases labour efficiency, factor mobility and specialization in occupations and trade, and the supply of entreprenurship. All these features are urgently necessary for economic development since low level of knowledge leads to low level of human development which can in turn severely constrain economic development. Education is a factor which plays a crucial role in developing human capital. It is not only an important objective of development by itself but is also fundamental to the broader notion of expanded human capabilities. Educated manpower is a prerequisite for increase in productivity, because it enables absorption of new technology. Most of the debate therefore relating to human capital, focuses around issues relating to the demand for and supply of education and its impact on the expansion of the economy. Though there are many non-market factors which affect the amount of schooling that person receives yet demand and supply occupy the most significant role. On the demand side one of the most important influences on the amount of schooling that an individual desires is the greater prospects of earning more income through future modern sector employment. In other words, the family's private benefits of education, is the most important determinant of the demand for education. Demand for education is thus in reality a derived demand for high wage employment opportunities in modern sector. The employment avenues particularly in less developing countries is determined by the individual's educational level. Consequently, demand for education is not for its intrinsic value, but because it is the only means of securing modern sector employment. Building of human capital through education is also determined to a large extent on the supply side by the quantity and quality of schooling and institutions of higher education, since it is the amount of education that is demanded that largely determines the supply.

Development of human resources through educational opportunities has therefore contributed to aggregate economic growth by creating a more productive labour force and endowing it with increased knowledge and skills. Education may, thereby, expand job opportunities, both directly as well as indirectly. Human resources can also be created through education, by training leaders, who can undertake the challenges of growth and development. Education also removes the various types of social and cultural impediments to modern strategy of growth. Though alternative forms of investment in the economy can generate greater growth, yet this does not reduce the important contributions, noneconomic as well as economic that development of human resources can result from education.

However, backward regions in less developing countries, such as north eastern region face double-layers of challenges to impart education in an attempt to develop its human resources. Firstly they belong to the whole nation, which already has its own challenges and problems of educational development. In 1990, India had an average of four years of schooling per worker as against eight years in developed countries. Secondly, being a backward region of a less developed nation it has numerous problems of its own nature. All these make achieving the goals of educational development much more difficult in such regions.

Records have revealed that the last 50 years have witnessed tremendous progress in education all over the world, with the progress being much more significant in the developing nations than in the developed ones. However, on the whole, record of educational achievement is much better in the high income nations than in the low income nations (HDR 1995). With higher income, people and governments can afford to spend more on education, resulting in higher productivity, which in turn gives rise to higher income level. At the same time evidence has shown that as normal goods, people do not spend more on education as income rises, as would have been expected.

Therefore, investment in children's education do not rise in proportion to rise in income. However, education particularly of the lower income group, enable them to make, the best use of economic opportunities. It is due to all these factors that, the new development paradigm has assigned tremendous importance to the role of education.

The role of education has aptly being emphasized by the proponents of new development economics, particularly for developing nations. In such nations, the initial stock of knowledge about the existing system is small to begin with, and the rate of economic progress is directly related to the increase in knowledge about the dynamics of growth (Naqvi : 2002). This very reality about the role of education for developing nations and the change that occurs in people's perception of this very reality due to development process has been fully taken into consideration by the advocates of development economics. New-classical economists however, failed to consider such issues having relevance to the common man.

Educational achievement has not only been extremely uneven throughout India, but so far government efforts in this regard left a lot to be desired. Though free and compulsory education till the age of 14 was one of the directive principles of the constitution, yet the measures adopted to achieve the goal was minimal. The idea of compulsory education has nowhere being implemented in India. Dreze and Sen (1995) have therefore postulated while expressing their views in this regard, that post-independence educational policy in India has been rather lamentable and suffered from numerous inconsistencies and contradictions like (i) confusion of objectives (ii) inconsistencies between stated goals and actual policy and (iii) specific contradiction between stated goals and resource allocation.

It is in this light that the present work will seek to examine in details the educational scenario of the various north eastern states of India. The study will attempt to analyse the scenario not only from the macro-view point of the state as a whole but also for the individual districts as well. Apart from this, macro-level analysis both for inter state and inter district level may often conceal crucial reality of the problem relating to diverse ethnic religious or social groups. The better performance of a small group of a region or state may convey a satisfactory average for the whole state or region. Consequently, when policy actions are adopted, the deprived sections may have a tendency to be pushed further into the peripherial level of their performance, since they are left out of the purview of the special treatment that is necessary for them. These sections of the population may not be aware (due to lack of education) of the facilities that are being offered to them. This results in the better off sections of the society ending up in enjoying major share of the various incentives and facilities. All these features may actually further widen the inter-group gap of educational achievement in the state. Another important feature of the study of literacy and the impact of public action, in this regard, is the spatial aspect. This aspect of analysis of educational achievement has received rather scant attention from both the researchers as well as by the policy makers. Benefits of public action is often confined to the central places or the core areas of development. The peripherial areas are often overlooked so that a wide gap in educational achievement may exist between the centre and the periphery. This may result in unbalanced development in education across the same state, though macro level data, may conceal much of these vital information. Consequently all these features will be examined from the point of view of not only rural and urban divide, but also from the point of view of the district with the state capital and the peripherial districts as well.

It is with this aim in view that the present study will examine the human resource development based on the various indicators of education across various ethnic social and economic groups of the various states of the region.

Methodology of the Study

For the purpose of the present study we have relied mostly on primary data. Data for the study have been collected from the six states of the north-eastern region. These states are Assam, Meghalaya, Mizoram, Nagaland, Arunachal Pradesh and Tripura. Data could not be collected from Manipur, due to the socio-economic turmoil of the state, which has made travelling to the state and collection of data extremely difficult. Data for the remaining states have been collected following the purposive multi-stage stratified sampling method. First tier in the process consisted of the selection of twenty percent of the districts, and the second consisted of the selection of twenty-percent blocks from the districts. From these blocks, we have taken twenty villages/towns, both in the rural as well as urban areas. From each of these villages/towns we have chosen twenty households in a purposive manner. Interview was then conducted through questionnaire method, and the requisite information derived.

District-wise analysis of Literacy Rate in North-East India

Literacy in Assam : Analysis of the data obtained through our sample survey for the six districts of Assam, namely Cachar, Karimganj, Kamrup, Jorhat, Barpeta and N. C. Hills, reveals that Kamrup and Jorhat districts achieved record literacy rates which is much higher than the state average. N. C. Hills and Cachar districts follow the trend of the state average but all the other districts fall much below the state average. Male literacy in all the districts is higher than the female literacy as is the experience in the entire country, with literacy rates in urban areas for all categories recording better rates than rural areas. This is not only due to better facilities in urban centres, but also due to the fact that demand for education is higher in urban areas. Existence of gender disparity in education is observed in both urban and rural areas with the latter experiencing a greater disparity. However, on the whole the disparity is lower than the all India figures. Lower educational status and greater degree of gender disparity in the rural areas is surely due to limited job opportunities coupled with inadequate facilities, but definitely not due to the lack of interest or desire for education.

Another feature that emerges from the analysis of our data of Assam on literacy rate is that district of Kamrup with the state capital has the highest literacy rate, both for the state as a whole, as well as for rural and urban sectors. This is also true both for male as well as female literacy rate, which are all higher in Kamrup district. This may imply that fruits of development and all other benefits are mostly concentrated in the core areas and declines as one goes to the peripherial areas. It also implies that demand for education is much higher in the core areas, since job opportunities, due to greater concentration of economic activities are also higher in such areas and diminishes towards the peripheral areas. Urban areas are therefore characterized by greater scope for human resource development both from the demand and the supply side. Such scope however diminishes as one moves towards the periphery.

Among the other districts of Assam, Barpeta is the worst performer in literacy with respect to both male and female literacy as well as rural and urban divide. Wide diversity is observed in terms of literacy even within the state itself. Assam being the largest state in the region, variation ranges between 68 percent in Kamrup district to only 50 per cent in Barpeta district. The range is 50.9 per cent to 79.9 per cent between rural and urban areas of the state. These wide variations are not only a product of differences in the level of effectiveness and implementation of public action, but also highlights the necessity of formulating public action in accordance with the specific problems of the particular area concerned.

Literacy in Mizoram : The state of Mizoram is one of the most literate states not only in the region but in the whole country as well, preceeded only by Kerala. In terms of our sample survey, it is revealed that Aizawl district has a literacy rate of 89.5 per cent and Chintuipui district has a literacy of 80.4 percent. Both these figures are much higher than the Indian average of literacy as well as the average of the north eastern region in terms of our sample survey figure. Both the districts surveyed by us also record extremely high figures both for male and female literacy as well. Even in the rural sectors of both the district, literacy rate in general as well as taken separately for males and females is much higher than the all India average.

A certain degree of gender disparity is observed even in the case of this state though the disparity is much lower, not only in both the districts but also between urban and rural areas, in comparison to all other states. In fact, in urban sectors of both the districts, gender disparity in terms of female male ratio of literacy rate is only 928. However, though the state presents a highly satisfactory picture of literacy rate yet the marginal gulf does exist even in case of this well performed state. Aizawl, the district with the state capital does much better, than the peripherial one of Chintuipui district.

The highly satisfactory overall performance in terms of education of this state may be attributed to many factors. One of the most crucial may be the role of the Christian missionaries in the spread of education for over 100 years. The multiplier effect of the initial years of education has worked itself out over all these years, through inter-generational effect, resulting in one of the best record of educational achievement in the whole country. High literacy rate increases the ability of the people of the state to make use of economic and social opportunities. The record of high literacy rate has been witnessed for many decades. Consequently, economic reforms could have been highly successful in Mizoram with a strong educational base like the South East Asian nations, which was not possible in the rest of India. The people of the region therefore has tremendous opportunities for raising the overall development of the state through its extremely rich human resource base.

Literacy in Nagaland : Performance of Nagaland is slightly lower than the all India performance as well as the average of the region, though wide variation is observed even within the state also. Even in case of this state we observe the centre-periphery relations between the core and the other districts. Existence of gender disparity is also present here, though it is considerably less in case of urban sectors. There is therefore considerable evidence to suggest that there is immense scope to raise the human resource base of the state in a planned way keeping the developmental needs of the state in mind.

Literacy in Tripura : Literacy rate in Tripura is marginally higher than the all India level, as well as the average literacy of the region. Even female literacy rate is higher in Tripura, than the all India average, though the existence of gender disparity is observed even in this state, which declines to some extent in the urban sectors. Tripura, therefore, seems to have the potential of human resource base, which only needs to be capitalized adequately for economic development through proper planning.

The centre periphery relation between the district is less acute in Tripura in comparison to other states of the region, though its existence is not ruled out totally.

The human resource base of the state has improved in a rather impressive manner over the past few years. The reasons for the improved performance may be attributed to factors, which differ from the performance of the other hill states. The state has not witnessed any long history of the work of the Christian missionaries for the spread of education as is witnessed in the other hill states. Perhaps strong public action and political commitment might have played a greater role in a rise of literacy in the state. However, the strong social infrastructure has not resulted in any commensurate degree of economic development. However the state certainly has a greater opportunity like Mizoram, unlike the other states of the region, to use education to develop skill centred industries, as is the case in certain other parts of India. These are certainly encouraging indicators, both for the state of Tripura and Mizoram. However even in these two states and particularly in Mizoram the wide inequalities that mark the performance of the rural and urban areas, may however act as a barrier to economic development in the years to come. The distribution of the benefits of economic development and social opportunities may also be distributed unequally.

Literacy in Meghalaya : The literacy rate in Meghalaya is higher than the average all India literacy rate and also that of the region as a whole. The performance of the rural sectors however is better in comparison to other states of the region. Presence of considerable amount of gender disparity both in urban as well as rural sector is evident, notwithstanding the fact that the state has a matrileanial system. Like Mizoram, Meghalaya too has experienced the role of the Christian missionaries for the spread of education, due to which the state records high literacy rate. Like other north eastern states, in Meghalaya too, the benefits of rich human resource base could not be utilised for economic development of the state. Therefore, more needs to be done by way of public action in the state to synchronize human resource development and economic development. Attention also needs to be given to the wide diversity that makes the performance between the rural and urban sectors of the various districts of the state. The literacy rate between rural and urban areas of East Khasi Hills ranges between 60 to 78.1 percent; while in East Garo Hills it ranges between 56.3 to 71.3 percent. Similar wide variation of 15 to 20 percent is witnessed for male and female literacy. Such wide variation not only reveals the insignificance of the state average, but also focusses attention to the insignificance of uniform public policies for rural and urban areas of the state. More concerted efforts need to be directed towards rural areas, the absence of which will not sustain any long term growth in the state.

Literacy in Arunachal Pradesh : The state has the lowest record of literacy rate in the whole region and is also one of the worst performer in the whole country with a literacy rate of only 39.54 percent in terms of our sample survey. Gender disparity in the state too is one of the highest in the whole region, which does not improve much even in case of urban areas, unlike the other states. Out of the two districts surveyed, the performance of Tirap district is the worst, with respect to all the indicators of literacy. The literacy rate of Tirap district reveals that 70 per cent of the females and 65 per cent of the males in the rural sector of the district are still illiterate, which improve only marginally in the urban sector of the district. Even in the core district where the state capital is located 68 per cent of the female population and 56 percent of the male population approximately are illiterate.

All these features relating to educational achievement of the state reveal that the various types of programmes undertaken for literacy campaign have not spread in the state, perhaps due to its peripherial location. This could be a possible explanatory factor behind the low literacy rate in the state, since the district of Tirap which is at the further peripherial level from the point of view of the core district of Itanagar, has a worse record. The district therefore suffers from various layers of negligence, firstly because it belongs to the periphery of the state and secondly the state itself is located at a peripherial zone of the already peripherial north-eastern region.

The educational scenario of the various states of the region therefore reveal that no two states can be treated at par, due to the wide difference in the degree and nature of performance and the factors responsible for the same. The variation in the performance between the states of Mizoram and Arunachal Pradesh is almost 45 percent, which increases to 50 per cent when we consider the best performing district of Mizoram and the worst performing district of Arunachal Pradesh. The contrast between these two states should be of particular interest for policy-makers, because nature and intensity of policies in Mizoram cannot be identical with Arunachal Pradesh. Consequently to treat the entire north-eastern region, as a homogeneous unit, as is the experience when policies are thrust from above, would only result in accentuating the problem of variation and differences of social and economic opportunities even further. In fact, population of Mizoram judging by their present performance can expect to be 50 times more capable and thereby expect to avail of social and economic opportunities by 50 times more than the population of Arunachal Pradesh.

Taking an overall view of the north-eastern region, what therefore transpires is that among the various states of north east for which we have been able to conduct the sample survey, states of Mizoram, Meghalaya and Tripura witness a literacy rate, which is higher than the all India average, whereas the remaining states of Assam, Nagaland and Arunachal Pradesh records lower literacy rate than the all India figures. Among these states, Mizoram is the best performer, whereas Arunachal Pradesh is the worst performer. Aizawl district of Mizoram and Tirap district of Arunachal Pradesh respectively has the best and the worst literacy records. Among the 16 districts, surveyed by us female literacy of 78 percent is the highest in Aizawl district and lowest in Itanager districts with only 32.35 percent. Gender disparity is the highest in Itanagar district of Arunachal Pradesh and the lowest in Chintuipui district of Mizoram. Even in the rural as well as in the urban sector, highest and lowest literacy rate is recorded respectively by Aizawl district of Mizoram and Tirap district of Arunachal Pradesh.

What therefore should be of concern for the purpose of public action is that, the general policy for the spread of literacy as is common in the rest of the country or even the other states of the region, cannot be applied with the same expected results in Arunachal Pradesh particularly Tirap district. In fact, though both Tirap district of Arunachal Pradesh as well as Aizawl district of Mizoram belong to the same region, there is a wide gulf between the two districts in terms of literacy rate. The former can be classified under the "low income countries", and the later under the "high income countries" in terms of the UNDP classification of nations. Therefore what is of relevance from our perspective is that the north-eastern region cannot be treated as a homogeneous unit for the purpose of public action, in view of its heterogeneous features. It is a homogeneous region as far as its geographical continuity is concerned but for all purpose of economic development and development of human resource, every individual part of the region deserves a unique treatment.

Enrolment rate as a determinant of literacy rate

In a formal system of education, enrolment is a necessary condition, but not a sufficient one for attaining literacy. Higher enrolment leads to higher literacy, provided it is not neutralized by higher drop out rates. Therefore enrolment rate (ER) is an important method of evaluating the educational status of a society. Article 45 of the Indian Constitution urges the states to provide free and compulsory education to all up to the age of 14 by 1960. This was indeed an ambitious goal, which could not be achieved. The means of achieving this objective was highly inadequate and consequently a large number of children up to the age of 14 have still not enrolled themselves in school. Even in 1986-87, nearly half of the rural children in the 6-11 years age group had never been enrolled at all. The revised National Policy on Education, 1992, only reiterated the earlier goal that it shall be ensured that free and compulsory education of satisfactory quality is provided to all children, upto 14 years before we enter the twenty-first century." The policy attempted to "adopt an array of meticulously formulated strategies based on micro-planning to ensure children's retention at school." However, once again the policy did not take any practical steps that would make the so-called 'resolved' a reality (Dreze & Sen : 2003). As a result even now we have not attained the goal of universal education for all children till 14 years of age. The lack of commitment of the government in this respect is evident from declining trend of public expenditure in education (Sengupta : 1998). This tendency has adversely affected provision of basic infrastructural school facilities, preventing the goal of universalisation of primary education. These facilities consisted of adequate pupil-teacher ratio, pupil-classroom ratio, basic teaching aids, building provision of essential services such as drinking water and sanitation facilities. The supply side factors relating to universalisation of education however varies from one state to another and from one region to another, which in turn determines the percentage of enrolment of children at elementary level of education.

From the point of view of demand side, crucial factors that determine enrolment of children in primary education is parental education. Educated parents understand the importance of sending their children to school and thereby motivate their children. The reverse is the experience with children who belong to families where education of parents is low. More important than parents education, is the mothers' education which has a positive effect in raising the enrolment rate. This is because female education has long run secondary effect. Type of occupation of the parents is another important factor determining the extent of enrolment. For instance, for parents engaged in the agricultural sector with low income level, education of children may not receive much of a priority. For similar reasons, where number of siblings in the family is large, ER may go down, particularly among the lower income group, due to sheer financial inadequacy. Female education is more adversely affected under such circumstances. Enrolment rate is also determined by the religious as well as socio-economic groups and the rural urban divide.

Enrolment Rate in North East India

Enrolment rate (E R) for our purpose is defined as the proportion of children in the age group of 6-14 years who have at any time enrolled in the school.

Variations in ER across different socio-economic linguistic ethnic and religious groups is made here in an attempt to identify the factors that determine enrolment rate in the region. The study reveals that enrolment rate in north eastern region has a definite relationship with the extent of educational attainment by the concerned state. Mizoram with 71.07 percent enrolment has the best figure in the whole region and it is also the state with highest literacy rate. In contrast, Arunachal Pradesh with the lowest literacy rate also has the lowest enrolment rate of only 42.86 per cent. This leads us to believe that high literacy rate may lead to high enrolment rate. The correlation between enrolment rate and literacy rate for the region as a whole, works out to be ·626. Enrolment rate for the region on the whole, is however lower than the all-India figure. Perhaps the difficult and inaccessible terrain makes accessibility to schools extremely difficult, resulting in lowering the average enrolment rate. Such an experience is more relevant for the far flung and inaccessible areas of Arunachal Pradesh. Though we have not explored this aspect of infrastructural facilities, yet it is quite possible, that lack of infrastructural facilities may be another reason for low enrolment rate. The often cited excuse that Indian parents have very little interest in the education of their children, is disproved by the high rate of parental literacy and enrolment rate among most religious and social groups of the north-eastern region. According to Dreze and Sen (2003), such opinions find a convenient rationalisation for the failure of most states to achieve universal elementary education. Sen opines that an overwhelming majority of Indian parents even among deprived sections of the population attach great importance to the education of their children. Only 3 percent of parents were opposed to compulsory education at the primary level.

Examining the enrolment across different social groups, it is revealed that on the whole the ST category of the population has a relatively high enrolment rate in most states of the region. This is true for states of Mizoram, Nagaland and Meghalaya, where enrolment rate among ST population exceeds the enrolment rate of the general category of the population. Highest enrolment rate of 75 per cent among the general category population is recorded only in Tripura. A striking feature is that the gap in the enrolment rate among the various social groups is very insignificant. Unlike the rest of India, the enrolment rate of the schedule caste, is not the lowest among the social groups. It may therefore, be conceded that there is very little discrimination on the basis of caste in the region. The ER of schedule caste group in some cases is higher than even the other social groups.

The contention that enrolment rate is determined by the literacy rate, is further evident by the rank correlation coefficient between enrolment rate of various social groups and their parental literacy rate, revealing the high degree of positive correlation between the two. It is the highest among the S.C. group, being as high as ·980, followed by ·800 for the ST group to ·620 for the general category. Parental education therefore seems to have a very significant impact on enrolment rate particularly among the deprived sections. This is true not only for north east India but for other parts of the country as well. The close relationship between adult literacy and enrolment rate is also supported by studies on Andhra Pradesh, which reveals the positive impact of adult literacy on enrolment rate.

What is even more interesting is that female literacy has a high degree of positive correlation with enrolment rate, which is highest among SC group, beings high as ·971. This is followed by ·819 among ST and ·620 among the general category. This finding reveals that if mothers and other female members of the family or society are literate, it can definitely have a direct as well as indirect impact on enrolment rate. Parental literacy rate and female literacy rate has greater impact on enrolment rate particularly for those groups who are either second or third generation learners, rather than for those who are several generation learners.

Enrolment rate by religious groups reveal that Christians perform better than all the other religious groups in Mizoram, Nagaland and Meghalaya. Record of the Hindu group is better than the other groups in the other three states dominated by this group. Demographic pattern on religious lives therefore appears to have a definite impact on ER. The enrolment rate 75.7 percent, the highest in the region, is witnessed by the Hindu group of Tripura. This is followed by the Christians of Mizoram, recording on enrolment rate of 72.85 percent. Muslims among all the religious groups record the lowest enrolment rate like the rest of India, though percentage of enrolment rate here is much higher than the all India figure. Perhaps the high literacy and enrolment of other groups might have had a positive demonstration effect in determining the enrolment rate even among the normally educationally backward group as considered in the rest of the country.

The worst performer in the region are the Buddhist religious groups, with only 40 percent enrolment rate found mostly in Arunachal Pradesh again leading us to conclude that demographic pattern of religion affects the ER. However, all groups, irrespective of their religion in the state record a very low literacy and enrolment rate.

The correlation between literacy rate and enrolment rate has also being worked out for different religious groups, in order to further substantiate our conclusion. The correlation coefficient of ·989 is the highest among the Christians revealing that education has resulted in enlighting this group with a consequent highest record of enrolment rate. The Hindu community also witnesses a high correlation coefficient of ·779. However, the coefficient is as low as ·612 among the Muslim community. All these findings reiterate our earlier hypothesis that literacy of the parents have favourable influence on enrolment rate, particularly as far as demand side of education is concerned.

An interesting feature relating to enrolment rate relates to gender disparity. Girls always seem to have a lower enrolment rate in comparison to boys, since investment in female education is generally considered as unremunarative investment. Again Dreze and Sen (2003) opine that parental commitment to female education is still rather inadequate in many areas. According to PROBE survey, 10 percent of the parents in BIMARU states still consider female education to be of no relevance. Practical commitment to female education even among those who consider female education as important is not very strong. Recognition of female education as a social issue is of recent origin. The authors further opine that educational aspirations are not independent of the opportunities that people have. Attitude towards female education is strongly influenced by cultural norms, role models, public discussions and related factors. Schooling decisions have significant social and religious dimensions, all of which have become clearly evident from our above analysis.

There is not much significant gender disparity among the various social groups. Only the groups considered as other backward class (OBC) in Karimganj district and SC's in Cachar district have a proportionately high gender disparity, though it is much lower than the all India scenario. It needs to be mentioned that enrolment rate of female exceeds that of males among the general category in Cachar district of Assam and enrolment rate is almost equal for the both males and females among the OBC's of the same district. However, low gender disparity is not related to high level of female literacy. Even in districts with low female literacy among some of the social groups, gender disparity in enrolment rate is low. This trend may imply that female education is not pushed to the backstage and given a secondary importance as in the rest of the country, resulting in a high enrolment rate among females, but due to poverty or other reasons girl students have a low retention rate.

Income is another important determinant of enrolment rate, because children belong to families of lower income group are not sent to school since (i) investment in children's education do not get priority and (ii) children have often to supplement family income, which prevents them from going to school. We have therefore attempted to examine enrolment rate of various income groups. Enrolment rate for all the districts reveal a clear rising trend, with a rise in income group, though there is considerable variation in percentage of enrolment rate across different income groups of the various states. The highest income group of Cachar district of Assam and Aizawl district of Mizoram, record the highest enrolment rate of 96.4 percent. In contrast, enrolment rate of 52.1 percent is the lowest among the lowest income group of Tirap district of Arunachal Pradesh. At the theoretical level therefore, it is revealed that economic prosperity has a positive impact on enrolment rate because poor economic condition compels households to keep their children away from school as the opportunity cost of time, (for supplementing household income) of going to school is very high for such people. Apart from this presence of children at home too is important otherwise parents will not be able to devote fully to wage employment. Consequently, lower income plays a more dominant role for ER in poor and backward district, where farm labour and wage employment are the major source of income.

Just as occupational structure has a definite relation with literacy rate, similary occupational pattern has a definite influence on enrolment rate. Children belonging to parents of agricultural sector of lower income group, may have lower enrolment rate, since the children are engaged in the fields along with their parents. Education therefore may not confer any direct benefit to such occupations and hence demand for education is not high. As against this, enrolment rate among children of parents engaged in business and service sector is high since education for them means higher income or better jobs and hence demand for education is high. Children of parents who are engaged as wage-earners or petty or irregular jobs, also have lower enrolment rate. The result of all these experiences is the emergence of a clear trend of enrolment which is discerned in all the sample districts of the various states of the region. Consequently enrolment is the highest among children of parents belonging to the service sector, denoting thereby that education is considered to be the main factor behind their employment and source of income. It declines for children whose parents are engaged in the manufacturing sector or small scale business or trade. Enrolment rate is the lowest among children of parents engaged as wage earners farm labour or petty jobs, implying that utility of education for such people is the lowest as they expect that their children will take up the type of jobs which they themselves perform. Such jobs do not require any education so that demand for education from such section is low. On the demand sides therefore, priority of education vary directly with the types of occupation of the parents. All these features, therefore, have important bearing on the formation of human resource of a region or place.

From the above analysis the factors that assume crucial significance, in determining the enrolment rate are (a) general literacy rate (b) female literacy rate (c) income level (d) occupational structure. However, among all the determinants, literacy rate in general and female literacy emerge as the most crucial determinants in terms of our earlier analysis. To discern the exact quantitative relationship among these variables, using enrolment rate as dependent variable and literacy rate and female literacy as independent variables, we have used regression model of the type:

$$ER = a + b\,lit + c\,lit_f$$

Where ER = enrolment rate
lit = general literacy rate
lit_f = female literacy rate

The above model has been examined for all the social and religious groups of the entire region in an attempt to know the impact of the various determinants of enrolment rate across different communities. The estimated results of the models tested for the north east region as a whole and for different religious and social groups/yield the following results:

$$ER = a + b\ lit + c\ lit_F$$

	a	b	c	R^2	F
N.E. Region	62.362	1.997	–2.163	.162	1.254
	(4.737)	(1.382)	(–1.496)		
Hindus	15.573	1.951	2.759	.772	5.069
	(.981)	(2.091)	(1.974)		
Christians	1.758	1.859	.760	.978	65.27
	(.379)	(2.074)	(1.82)		
Muslims	128.673	–.665	.478	.099	.219
	(1.058)	(–.612)	(.440)		
Schedule Tribe	18.163	.629	1.442	.678	13.156
	(1.02)	(2.255)	(2.586)		
Schedule caste	24.531	1.053	–.074	.960	47.921
	(6.633)	(1.177)	(–.082)		
General Category	59.245	6.962	7.693	.923	18.092
	(5.461)	(3.706)	(4.096)		

Perusual of the estimated results of the regression model reveals that the model is not acceptable for the region as a whole. Explanatory power of the variable judged by the value of R^2 is not only extremely weak but the model cannot be accepted either on statistical or theoretical grounds. This may lead one to conclude that the model using general literacy rate and female literacy is not acceptable for the region. However, exploring the relationship at the micro level for the various religious and social groups disproves our initial conclusion.

Examining the model across different religious groups, it is revealed that 98 percent and 77 per cent of the relationship is explained by the model in case of Christian and Hindu community respectively. However, explanatory power of the variable is extremely weak in case of the Muslim community and the coefficients of the independent variables are not statistically significant. It is therefore, evident that model is not applicable in case of the Muslim community. This may imply that enrolment rate for this community may be explained by some other socio-economic variables, and neither the literacy rate in general or female literacy has much of an impact on enrolment rate. However, the same is not true with respect of the Hindu and the Christian community for whom the model is acceptable since the coefficients of literacy rate and female literacy are theoretically satisfactory and statistically significant.

Examining the model for the various social groups, it is revealed that explanatory power of the model ranges between 96-68 percent. Though it is the highest in case of the schedule caste, yet the coefficient for female literacy is neither statistically nor theoretically significant due to which the model is rejected in their case. Though education has a greater impact particularly for the new generation learners but for the schedule caste group of the region education is a common feature among them for many generations and thereby occupational structure and economic prosperity might have a greater role to play in determining enrolment rate. The model is acceptable for both the schedule tribe as well as the general category group and the fit is best in case of the later group.

Conclusion

It may therefore be concluded that taking an overall view, though it may seem that education do not have much of an impact on enrolment rate, but examination of data for micro-groups reveals that for most groups education can influence the enrolment rate, though significant inter group variation is worth noting.

The human resource potential of the north eastern states of India therefore not only emerges to be immensely diverse but reveals that the positive achievements of some of the states in the region can be comparable to better performing states like Kerala. In contrast we have the experience of Arunachal Pradesh and some districts of Assam whose educational performance is comparable to the BIMARU states. However the factors determining the present scenario of human resource in the north eastern states, whether in the best performing or worst performing states are different from the rest of India. Public action relating to any economic problem is shaped by the gravity of the determinants leading to the prevaling situation. Consequently public action needed to improve human resources or gear them for economic development needs to be different from the rest of the country. States of the north-east India which are often left out of the main focus of any serious discussion, present unique picture of lower gender disparity and almost a total absence of any kind of social discrimination in education in comparison to all India scenario. Even some religious minorities who normally perform poorly at the all India level, do much better in the north-eastern states, factors which need to be highlighted in matters of any serious work on north-east and for public action as well. It is therefore, evident that the north-eastern states on the whole are doing quite well as far as development of human resources are concerned. Public action therefore has to be focused more towards channelizing these resources for economic uplift of the region.

REFERENCES

Dreze and Sen (2003) *India Development and Participation*, OUP. New Delhi.

_______________(1995) *Indian Economic Development and Social Opportunities*, OUP. New Delhi.

Naqvi, S. (2002) : *Development Economics—Nature and Significance,* Sage Publications, New Delhi.

Sengupta K. (1998) : "Trends of Educational Expenditure and its Impact on the Indian Economy", in *Indian Economy after 50 years of Independence Experience and Challenges* , ed., D.K. Das, Deep and Deep Publication, New Delhi.

UNDP, (1995) : *Human Development Report,* Oxford University Press.

6

ROLE OF EDUCATION IN HUMAN DEVELOPMENT IN NAGALAND

– *Subhendu Dutta*

Economic development of a country necessitates the development of its manpower. Besides the development of physical resource, there is need to develop human resources, which play a pivotal role in the overall development of a country or a region. Skilled human beings are required to exploit the physical resources of a country in an optimum manner. Thus human development is of utmost importance, particularly when the country is still in the early phases of development. UNDP has defined human development as a process of enlarging people's choices, as well as raising the level of well-being. It recognises the choice to lead a long and healthy life, the choice to acquire knowledge and be educated, and to have access to resources needed for a decent level of living as the three most critical and socially valuable choices. It is thus quite apparent that human development will be triggered when people of that country have been enjoying a decent life, are well-educated and technically trained, when they have access to good medical facilities and balanced diet. Realization of all the above will therefore increase one's welfare. However, we cannot deny the fact that all these prescribed indicators of human development in a country are very intimately related to one key indicator, that is, education. Its role in human and hence economic development is unquestionable. Evidence show that an educated society has boundless power to overcome various hindrances to economic development. In fact, development of human resources can be effected by a campaign of mass literacy. Sen opined that primary education should be treated as a fundamental right of a citizen. He has put emphasis on the role of education in providing vertical mobility to the poor to acquire better skills and training so as to become suitable for better jobs. In this sense, education helps to improve efficiency of labour, create entitlement about rights and this becomes a vehicle to the reduction of poverty. Education ensures the best means to attain the goal of equality of opportunity in the society. "The objectives of education are twofold : (i) to rationalize and modernize the attitudes of those who receive education and in turn, to inculcate and nurture such attitudes among the rest of the society through the "educated" ones, and (ii) to impart to the recipients of education the knowledge and skill together with the ability to acquire further knowledge and still better skill by their own efforts. The touchstone of the worth of an education system is in meeting these objectives. (Misra http://www.freewebs.com/nehu_economics/hrdner.pdf).

> "Education, in the present day context, is perhaps the single most important means for individuals to improve personal endowments, build capability levels, overcome constraints and, in the process, enlarge their available set of opportunities and choices for a sustained improvement in well-being. It is not only a means to enhance human capital, productivity and, hence, the compensation to labour, but it is equally important for enabling the process of acquisition, assimilation and communications of information and knowledge, all of which augment a person's quality of life. Education is important not merely as means to other ends, but it is

> an attribute that is valued in itself, by most individuals. More importantly, it is a critical invasive instrument for bringing about social, economic and political inclusion and a durable integration of people, particularly those 'excluded', from the mainstream of any society. The process of education and attainments thereof has an impact on all aspects of life. It captures capability of acquiring knowledge, communication, and participation in community life. It alters an individual's and even community's collective perceptions, aspirations, goals as well as the ability and the means to attain them. The level and spread of education has not only been an important precondition for sustained economic growth, both in the developed and the developing countries, but it has also played a critical facilitative role in the demographic, social and political transition of these societies. Creation, application and adaptation of new technologies; lower fertility, infant and child mortality rates; better nutritional, hygiene and health status of children, reproductive health and empowerment of women; social mobility and political freedom, all have visible linkages with educational attainments of people. It is, undoubtedly, a basic component of human development." (NHDR : 2001)

Further, "Economic development depends not only on the supply of the brute muscular power that human beings can apply to transformation of the non-human resources to more useful forms, but also on the skill embodied in the manpower applied to the production processes. Skill formation among the illiterate, though very important for economic development, has quite limited scope. Therefore, literacy and some extent of educational proficiency are of fundamental importance. Literacy among the females is of great importance, not only for participation in productive and civic activities, but also for rearing children for a better future (Misra: op.cit).

Improvements in educational attainments have customarily

been accompanied by improvement in health and longevity of the population and in their economic well-being. Educated people are likely to be more productive and hence better off. They are also likely to contribute more to a country's economic dynamics of a society towards equality in attainments and opportunities for its people. Though, the returns to education may vary across individuals, regions, level and nature of education, in general, they are significantly higher for poor developing areas than for the rich. Education is therefore, the best social investment, given the synergies and the positive externalities that it generates for people in their well-being. It is also a priority for countries seeking to develop and sustain their level and pace of development. The UNDP in its HDR 1990, pointed out, and rightly so, that literacy is a person's first step in learning and knowledge building and, therefore, literacy indicators were essential for any measurement of human development.

A number of studies confirmed a positive relationship between education and the level of economic development by way of human development. To quote the World Bank, "Developed countries with high literacy rates have tended to grow faster, even after allowances are made for differences in incomes and physical investment, and they have higher physical investment rates." It is also empirically true that increasing education by 6 years lifted economic growth rates by 39 per cent. Studies have shown that if a farmer had completed four years of elementary education, his/her productivity was on an average, 8.5 per cent higher than that of a farmer who had no education at all. In case of India there is evidence that adoption and spread of 'green revolution', in 1960s, was faster among the educated farmers. In industry, most evidence suggests that at enterprise level educated workers are more productive. More strikingly, the skill and knowledge intensive sectors have been the fastest growing service sector in India in recent years. If we look at the IT sector, we will find that a pool of technical humans have been produced in this sector - meeting both domestic and foreign demands of total stock of IT men. A study for 88 countries for the period 1960-63 and 1970-73 found that an increase in literacy from 20 per cent to 30 per cent were associated with an increase in real GDP of between 8 and 16 per cent. Another study of 37 middle- income and 29 low-income countries indicated that a 1 per cent difference in the primary enrolment ratios was associated with 0.035 per cent difference in per capita income growth rates (NHDR : 2001). Education increases equality as well. A study of 49 countries showed that about a fifth of income-inequality could be explained by educational inequality. Another study has shown that an increase in literacy rate from 10 to 60 per cent has ben associated with a 2.8 per cent increase in the income share for the poorest 40 per cent of the population. At lower levels of development, in some cases, expanding education could possibly increase inequality, but with development, education does seem to generally have an income levelling effect. The poor countries get much higher rates of return than the rich countries from investing in education. For the poorest countries, the highest returns are from primary education. For instance, in case of African countries the estimated rate of return on primary education was 26 per cent in comparison to 17 per cent for secondary education and 13 per cent for higher education. In case of India, as per one study, the private rate of return per year of education increases as the level of education increases up to the secondary level. The returns of primary education were rather low and, in general, returns, per year at secondary level were the highest. It was also seen that returns to women's education exceeded that of man at middle, secondary and higher secondary levels. (NHDR : 2001)

National Human Development Report has put together indicators and composite indices as laid down by the UNDP for human development in a country to evaluate development process in terms of 'ex-post outcomes' rather than only in terms of available 'means' or 'inputs.' The Report, recognizing the broad based consensus that exists on the three critical dimensions of well-being focused on identifying the various contextually relevant indicators on each of them. These dimensions or HDI of well-being are related to :

1. Longevity—the ability to live long and healthy life;
2. Edcuation—the ability to read, write and acquire knowledge; and
3. Command over resources—the ability to enjoy a decent standard of living and have a socially meaningful life.

In order to examine inter-state position on HRD, NHDR has introduced Development Radars for various Indian States. Development Radars are the diagrammatic representation of progress of states, separately for rural and urban areas, drawn on eight distinct social indicators for two points of time namely, early 1980s and early 1990s. The following indicators have been selected for the purpose highlighting each state's standing on human development:

1. Per capita consumption expenditure;
2. Incidence of poverty as depicted by the head count ratio;
3. Access to safe drinking water;
4. Proportion of households with *pucca* houses,
5. Literacy rate for the age group 7 years and above;
6. Intensity of formal education;
7. Life expectancy at age 1 and
8. Infant mortality rates.

Development Radars at a glance give a picture of attainments on the three critical dimensions of well-being (HDI) as well as highlight the progress in meeting the basic human needs of accessibility to safe drinking water and shelter in various Indian states.

The present chapter attempts to examine the extent of human development that has effected by way of education in the state of Nagaland, by studying the various specific indicators under the one broad heading - education, in order to bring true nature of human resource development taking place in the state in the recent years. An attempt is made for comparison of the state in this respect with other states in NER and also with India as a whole. The indicators such as literacy rate of the population, including, those for adults, females, the deprived and the backward, enrolment, attendance and dropout rates of the school going children or the girl child, or the proportion of population having higher and technical qualification, etc. have been used to measure the level of educational attainment in the state. The level of government participation in terms of expenditure on education has also been looked into. Indicators reflecting qualitative aspect of educational attainment are also, to some extent, dealt with.

Before we analyse the specific indicators reflecting the state's position on education front as a measure of HRD, it would be imperative to have a glance at the overall picture of human development in India as well as in various states of NER. In this connection it would also be helpful to supplement this with the Development Radars as prepared by NHDR for instant examination of inter-state differences on human development. As such the Development Radars of Nagaland is shown along with that of India as a whole. Development Radars for NE states of Manipur, Meghalaya, Mizoram, Nagaland, Tripura and Sikkim, show that the attainments on shelter and acessibility to safe water are relatively poor and not much progress seems to have taken place. At the national level, it can be seen that attainments in the human development indicators in urban areas are better than rural. The rural-urban gap for most indictors has, however, declined. Substantial gap remains to be covered in areas like per capita expenditure and poverty.

Table 6.1 shows that HDI value in 1981 was 0.328 and that of India as a whole was 0.302. In terms of ranking, Nagaland is 3rd in NER, Manipur and Mizoram being 1st and 2nd positions

Table 6.1
Human Development Index for the States of NEI - 1991

States/UTs	Rural		Urban		Combined		Gender Disparity index	
	Value	Rank	Value	Rank	Value	Rank	Value	Rank
Arunachal Pradesh	0.30	28	0.572	15	0.328	29	0.776	18
Assam	0.326	26	0.555	19	0.348	26	0.575	30
Manipur	0.503	7	0.618	12	0.536	09	0.815	03
Meghalaya	0.332	24	0.624	10	0.365	24	0.807	12
Mizorum	0.464	10	0.648	05	0.548	07	0.770	06
Nagaland	0.442	13	0.633	07	0.486	11	0.729	21
Tripura	0.368	20	0.551	20	0.389	22	0.531	29
All-India	0.340		0.511		0.381		0.676	

Source : National Human Development Report-2001.

respectively. Among all states in the country Nagaland ranks 20, whereas Manipur rating very high at 4th position. HDI values for rural areas indicate that Nagaland ranks 19th among all Indian states and in NER it is 3rd behind Manipur and Mizoram in that order. Urban ranking in terms of HDI for Nagaland is quite good in 1981, that is 8th, again maintaining the 3rd position in NER. Gender disparity index show that is 16th in the list in 1981, which however slid down to 21 in 1991. But there has been a significant improvement in HRD in Nagaland in 1991 as evident from the table that it saled to 11th position from 20th in 1981. Almost 50 per cent improvement of HRD in the state. The values being 0.328 and 0.486 respectively. In case of urban areas, it again gained one point and scaled to 7th position. Similar was the position for rural HDI ranking. During both the periods, the values for Nagaland were higher than the figures for India as whole.

Literacy Rate

Literacy rate is the proportion of literates to total population in age group 7 years and above (Census of India). It was merely 18.3 per cent (for the age group 5 years and above) in 1951, 43.6 per cent in 1981, and 52.2 per cent in 1991 in the country which has significantly increased in recent years. Table 6.2 reveals that literacy rate in Nagaland in 1981 was 50.28 per cent, in 1991 61.65 per cent and in 2001, it was 67 per cent. All these figures are higher than all India figures for the same periods. Within NER, Nagaland is placed fourth, the first being Mizoram. Nevertheless, Nagaland is ahead of Assam and Meghalya.

There has been a marked increase in literacy rate among females in Nagaland over the period 1981-2001. In 1981 female literacy was only 40.38 per cent which went up to 62 per cent in 2001.

There are, however, large inter-state variations in literacy rates in the NER itself. However, it is declining since 1981, though the disparities become more distinct if one takes into

Table.6.2
Literacy Rate in NE States-(1981-2001)

(Percentage)

States/UTs	1981			1991			2001		
	Male	Female	Persons	Male	Female	Persons	Male	Female	Persons
Arunachal Pradesh	35.12	14.02	25.55	51.45	26.69	41.59	64.07	44.24	54.74
Assam	—	—	—	61.87	43.03	52.89	71.93	56.03	64.28
Manipur	64.15	34.67	49.66	71.63	47.60	59.89	7.87	59.70	68.87
Meghalaya	46.65	37.17	42.05	53.12	44.85	49.10	66.14	60.41	63.31
Mizorum	79.36	68.61	74.26	85.61	78.60	82.27	90.69	86.13	88.49
Nagaland	58.58	40.38	50.28	67.62	54.75	61.65	71.77	61.92	67.11
Tripura	61.49	38.01	50.11	70.58	49.65	60.44	81.47	65.41	73.66
All-India	56.38	29.76	43.57	64.13	39.29	52.21	75.64	54.03	65.20

Source : National Human Development Report-2001

Note : 1. Census not held in Assam in 1981.

2. Literacy Rate is defined as the proportion of literates to the population in the age group 7+.

3. For Census 1981, Literacy rate was defined for the population 6+. To ensure comparability in this exercise it has been re-estimated for the population 7+.

account rural-urban differences or the differences between male and female literacy rates. The literacy rate in rural Nagaland increased from about 46 per cent in 1981 to 63 per cent in 2001. The corresponding rates in urban Nagaland were about 76 and 86 per cent, respectively. Thus, rural-urban gap has declined from about 30 to 23 percentage points. During this period, literacy rate for males in Nagaland increased from about 59 per cent, in 1981 to nearly 72 per cent in 2001-a very significant rise indeed. The corresponding change in female literacy rate has ben from around 40 per cent to 62 per cent. The decline in rural-urban gap from 30 to 23 percentage points was almost similar to that of gender gap in the same periods. Gender gap in Nagaland, in general and in case of rural areas interestingly, remained the same. In both cases it declined from 18 in 1981 to about 10 in 2001. Urban gender gap in the state in 1981 was about 9 which came down to 7 in 2001. As against the overall literacy rate of 61.65 per cent in 1991, literacy rate for Scheduled tribes was 60.59 per cent.

The disparities in male and female literacy rate among Scheduled Tribes were quite higher than those for the rest of the population. It is about 11.76 per cent in 1991, a slight decline from the 14.33 per cent in 1981.

Adult Literacy Rate

The adult literacy rate in India is defined as the proportion of literate population in age group 15 years and above. It also gives an indication of the stock of human capital in population. The proportion of adult literates in the population increased from about 41 per cent in 1981 to about 49 per cent in 1991 in the country.

The proportion of adult literates in the state increased from about 49 per cent in 1981 to about 59 per cent in 1991 and to 81 per cent in 1995-96. Adults literate in rural areas were 44 per cent, 55 per cent and 77 per cent respectively in these years. Thus there has been an improvement in case of adult literacy in the state. In urban areas, the percentages of adult literates during the same periods were 75 per cent, 82 per cent and 88 per cent respectively. There has been a considerable decline in gender gap from 21 in 1981 to 16 in 1991 and down to 11 in 1995-96.

Enrolment in Schools

The enrolment of children in schools depicts the current flow or the spread of education. The alternate measures for analyzing enrolment of children in schools are gross enrolment ratio, age-specific enrolment ratio, net enrolment ratio, dropout rates and school attendance rates, are relevant for capturing the flow aspect of the educational attainment of the population. Gross Enrolment Ratio refers to enrolment at a specified level of schooling, irrespective of the age of student enrolled, to the population of children in the age group expected to be at that level of schooling as per prevalent norms on school enrolments. Gross Enrolment Ratio for Class I-V (6-11 years) in 1999-2000 in the state was 90, 87.8 in 2000-01 and 85.2 in 2001-02. Thus gross enrolment ratio has declined over the years.

The girls enrolled in class I-V increased from about 44 per cent in 1978 to 48 per cent i.e, by 4 percentage points increase in 1993. For other classes enrolment ratio remained same over the period.

Age Specific Enrolment Ratio

It refers to percentage of children enrolled in a particular age group, irrespective of the level/class of enrolment, to the total population of children in that age group. A higher ratio on this measure implies a higher educational participation. However, it suffers from a limitation that it does not give the schooling level/ class at which the students are enrolled.

The age-specific enrolment ratio for age group 6-14 years remained same in Nagaland at about 58 per cent in both the years 1981 and 1991. For rural areas, it increased negligible from

54.9 per cent to 55.45 per cent while for urban areas the correponding ratios were 81.55 per cent and 74.6 per cent respectively. The ratio for boys decreased from 62.6 per cent in 1981 to 58.6 per cent in 1991. For girls, the ratio increased from 55.15 per cent in 1981 to 56.8 per cent in 1991. Thus, the rural-urban gap, as well as gender gap almost remained same during the period 1981 to 1991. A break up of age group 6-14 years into 6-10 yeas and 11-14 years shows that age-specific enrolment ratio is significantly lower in age group 6-10 years than in age group 11-14 years in 1991, a swell as in 1981.

Drop Out Rate

It is the percentage of students dropping out of class/classes in a given year. Along with students repeating a class, the drop out rate gives an indication about the wastage of school education and tends to undermine benefits of increased enrolments. Though, the drop out rate at national level for India has been declining, there is considerable regional disparity in the magnitude.

Drop-out ratios among children who are studying in class I-V in 1998-99 was 35.94 per cent, for class I-VIII 42.98 per cent and for class I-X it was 62.59 per cent in Nagaland. It is observed that larger number of students drop out by the time they reach class X. The average drop-out rates for class I-X for 1998-99 is 62.59 per cent, for 1981-82 it was 90.66 per cent and 76.53 per cent in 1992-93. Thus a significant decline is apparent in drop out of students going to classes I to X in the state. It is a good sign as it reflects higher rates of retention in school going children. Another important fact evident is that drop out rates in Nagaland in all these years was lower than that in other states of NER. The drop out rate has also not been higher for girls as is the case for India as a whole. It is only when the enrolled students are retained over successive classes that the indicator of enrolment becomes useful from the point of capturing the current educational progress in a society. It is this concern that makes it necessary to look at

Table 6.3
Age-specific Enrolment Ratio - Combined in NE States

(Percentage)

States/UTs	Age Group 6 to below 11 years						Age group 11 to below 14 years					
	1981			1991			1981			1991		
	Boys	Girls	Children	Boys	Girls	Children	Boys	Girls	Children	Boys	Girls	Children
Arunachal Pradesh	39.2	24.1	31.9	42.6	33.4	38.1	54.2	30.0	42.8	68.7	53.7	61.5
Assam	—	—	—	49.0	42.9	46.0	—	—	—	67.9	58.7	63.4
Manipur	55.1	46.1	50.7	50.2	46.0	48.1	76.2	58.4	67.4	75.7	68.0	71.9
Meghalaya	37.4	37.8	37.6	34.7	34.5	34.6	48.5	50.3	49.4	54.6	56.1	55.4
Mizorum	72.8	72.2	72.5	64.0	62.6	63.3	83.7	77.4	80.6	79.8	75.5	77.6
Nagaland	52.1	46.4	49.3	48.9	45.4	47.2	73.1	63.9	68.6	71.7	68.2	70.0
Tripura	57.0	49.1	53.2	55.1	49.6	52.4	68.0	53.5	60.9	78.0	68.3	73.2
All-India	55.3	38.5	47.2	56.6	45.4	51.2	62.0	36.7	50.0	71.1	52.2	62.1

Source : National Human Development Report - 2001

Note: Age-Specific Enrolment Ratio = (Estimated enrolment in an age group/Estimated child population in that age group) × 100

Table 6.4

Drop-out Rates in Classes I-X in NE States

(Percentage)

States/UTs	1981-82			1992-93			1998-99 (Provisional)		
	Boys	Girls	Children	Boys	Girls	Children	Boys	Girls	Children
Arunachal Pradesh	90.63	90.87	90.70	78.12	80.02	78.83	76.09	78.67	77.20
Assam	63.30	67.81	65.09	74.28	78.13	75.95	76.55	75.32	76.00
Manipur	88.01	88.75	88.33	74.57	74.45	74.52	76.35	76.74	76.54
Meghalaya	90.82	91.66	91.22	67.93	68.07	68.00	62.12	63.74	62.89
Mizorum	86.8	91.08	88.97	57.00	54.37	55.72	73.85	71.10	72.56
Nagaland	89.33	92.35	90.66	75.03	78.22	76.53	63.84	60.98	62.59
Tripura	84.95	86.53	85.59	81.72	83.16	82.36	79.94	83.95	81.78
All-India	79.44	86.81	82.33	70.00	77.32	72.93	65.44	70.22	67.44

Source : National Human Development Report - 2001.

Table 6.5
Intensity of formal Education - 1993 in NE States

(Years)

States/UTs	Rural			Urban			Combined		
	Boys	Girls	Children	Boys	Girls	Children	Boys	Girls	Children
Arunachal Pradesh	4.08	3.71	3.93	5.66	5.43	5.56	4.33	4.01	4.20
Assam	4.24	4.13	4.19	5.57	5.40	5.49	4.41	4.30	4.36
Manipur	4.40	4.32	4.36	5.63	5.50	5.57	4.80	4.72	4.76
Meghalaya	4.40	4.32	4.36	5.63	5.50	5.57	4.80	4.72	4.76
Mizorum	3.84	3.85	3.85	4.62	4.72	4.67	4.20	4.28	4.24
Nagaland	3.88	3.85	3.87	4.96	5.05	5.01	4.21	4.23	4.22
Tripura	4.23	4.01	4.13	5.75	5.66	5.71	4.50	4.32	4.42
All-India	4.41	3.99	4.25	5.63	5.36	5.51	4.77	4.46	4.64

Source : National Human Development Report-2001

Note : Intensity of formal education has been estimated as the weighted average of the enrolled students from Class I to Class XII (where weights being 1 for Class 1, 2 for class II and so on) to the total enrolment Classes I to Class XII.

indicators like the 'mean year of schooling' or for that matter "intensity of formal education.'

Intensity of Formal Education

This indicator is based on class-wise enrolment rates and it attempts to reflect current progress in spread of formal education among school going children. This indicator not only values education in early years of an individual's life (as it looks at children in the school going age-group but it lays importance on a structured formal system of education (unlike non-formal education like adult literacy) and, more importantly, weighs progressively the capacity of the education system to retain enrolled students over successive classes from class I to XII. As a result, it implicitly takes care of the drop out rates across all classes.

In Nagaland, the intensity of formal education was 3.71 years fro students enrolled in 1978. It increased to 4.22 years in 1993. It was lower for girls in 1978 in comparison to boys. For boys, it increased from 3.11 yeas in 1978 to 4.21 years in 1993, while for girls it increased from 3.59 years to 4.23 years. Thus, during this period gender gap declined from 0.22 to 0.02 years. In rural areas this decline was higher from 0.22 to 0.03 years, than in urban areas which were 0.25 in 1978 and 0.09 years in 1993. The rural-urban difference was significant in both years at 1.78 and 1.14 years respectively. In other words, intensity of formal education in 1978 for rural areas was about 66 per cent of urban areas rising significantly to about 77 per cent in 1993. The number of primary schools serving total population in the state has declined over the years from 13.71 per thousand population in 1982-83 to only 8.89 schools in 1992-93 and down to 6.8 in 1997-98. For upper primary, similar is the trend. At all India level, however, there has been a slight increase in the number of schools at both the levels. In other NE states, data indicate a declining trend, however, a marginal increase in the number in case of primary schools in Assam.

Policy Measures and Suggestions

In India, the responsibility of educational development and spread of literacy rests largely with state governments. The central government has also been taking initiatives, under its constitutional obligations, to supplement the efforts of state governments by meeting some critical gaps in public provisioning for literacy improvement, particularly in the educationally backward states. These efforts have taken the shape of an enabling policy framework - for instance, the National Education Policy 1986, and the more recent step of introducing the bill for making primary education compulsory in the parliament, as well as specific programmes including the Total Literacy Campaign, District Primary Education Programme (DPEP), Mahila Samakhya or the present initiative on Sarva Shiksha Abhiyan embodying some of these past programmes. (The Sarva Shiksha Abhiyan is a time-bound initiative of the central government, partnership with the states, the local governments and the community, to provide elementary education to all children in the age group 6-14 years by 2010. It recognizes the importance of community owned system organized in a mission mode for improving reach and performance of the school system).

Improving accessibility of children, in school going age group, to schools and increasing enrolment rates have been backed in some cases by visible measures to improve qualitative aspect of schooling. This has led to improvements in student retention rates (i.e., decline in drop out rates) in schools and, hence, better performance on educational indicators. However at state level, the proportion of children with access to primary school within the habitation or within a distance of half a kilometre slightly fell from 98 per cent in 1978 to 93 per cent in 1993, this proportion in case of access to upper primary schools (middle schools) — up to a distance of one kilometre — increased by about 6 percentage points from 57 per cent in 1978 to 63 per cent in 1993. A similar trend was noticeable in case of 'teacher-pupil ratio'— an indicator having a bearing on quality of education and, hence, on retention of enrolled children in schools. The ratio refers to number of students enrolled for every teacher appointed. This ratio has not changed significantly in the fifteen years between 1982-83 and 1997-98. During this period it remained same at 21 students in primary classes, increased from 15 to 19 students in middle classes and from 23 to 29 students per teacher for secondary classes. This ratio for primary school in 1999-2000 was 20. Thus, at both the national and state levels, the appointment of teachers kept pace with increasing enrolment in schools.

Public support by way of allocation of resources for creation and maintenance of education infrastructure has a direct bearing on some of these indicators. Over the period 1980-81 to 1998-99 'education expenditure ratio', i.e., the percentage of public expenditure on education to the total public expenditure has increased consistently at both central and state level. The ratio for Nagaland increased from 8.3 to 9.5 between 1980-81 and 1998-99. The increase in share of public expenditure on education to total public expenditure has also increased from about 7 per cent in1980-81 to 12 per cent in 1990-91. As total percentage of gross state domestic product, public spending on education and in the state and also national levels fell dramatically. It declined from about 84 per cent in 1980-81 to about 28 per cent in 1998-99. In recent years, in Nagaland, private expenditure on educational services has been increasing at a rapid rate, not only at primary levels but also at higher educational levels. This is due the government policy in favour of private participation which will not only open avenues for the unemployed but also help the government in reducing the burden on exchequer. This is evident from the growing presence of private and missionary schools from kindergarden level to vocational and professional colleges throughout the state. They have become important in bridging the gap between the demand and the supply of education in the society, both in terms of quantity and quality. In many instances, they are the result of specific demands of the market, for instance, institutions imparting computer literacy and other skills have proliferated like anything in recent years. Like other developed states of the country, one can easily access to almost all reputed institutions names providing computer education in the state. An important feature of the strategy in the state that has made rapid strides in raising the literacy rates, apart from improved enrolment rates of children in school going age group, relates to the success in bringing down the drop out rates and increasing participation of private individuals in imparting education. Innovative changes in curriculum made both by Nagaland Board of Secondary Education for school education and Nagaland University for higher education, including exposure to vocational training, flexibility in scheduling of school terms, particularly in rural areas, keeping in view the requirement of large segment of children who are, perpetually, called up to meet seasonal demand for labour in agriculture sector, and evening/night schools/colleges in urban areas, which is however now slowly picking up, have been seen to be helpful in improving enrolments and retaining children in schools for longer duration. There is a need to revolutionize the educational system in line with skill-generating curricula. The existing educational institutions will have to start technical and professional education programmes. For instance, a commerce student who passes out with a degree is not comfortable with various accounting packages available and frequently used in company. Education is still a one man show, playing leading role by the person who imparts it and no participation from the students' side. Such a defective and monotonous system of educational instructions used at all levels of education needs to be removed and a more interesting and workable way needs to be sorted out. An aspect of the current national policy focus in education that has a bearing on the future prospects of educational attainment for the society at large relates to the education of the girl child. The Approach to the Tenth Plan aims at bringing down gender gap in literacy by 50 per cent over the plan period in the country. Initiatives like the *Mahila Samakhyan* that focuses on creating a greater access to education, generates demand for education, build capacities and strengthen women's abilities to effectively participate in village level processes for educational development have to be pursued vigorously in different states having significant differential in male-female literacy rates. National Programe for Education of Girls at Elementary Level (NPEGEL) has been launched in 2003-04 for providing components for girls' education at elementary level under SSA will also help increasing the rate of enrolment of girls. Percentage of girls enrolled in various school stages over 1978 to 1993 indicates marginal increasing trend in the state. But for the class IX onwards the figures remained almost same.

The progress in the state in regard to educational development vis a vis human development reflects a healthy trend. Private participation in education is very high in Nagaland as compared to any other state in NER, at almost all levels of educational stages. Drop out rates have been falling along with the gender gap and rural urban differences. Technical education in IT sector specifically has been progressing at a fast pace due rapid rise in private institutions providing IT related education. Nevertheless, there is dearth of engineering and medical institutions in the state. The number of ITIs in Nagaland in 1997 was only 3 with seating capacity of 404. Another very important feature in Nagaland is excessive government spending on scholarships to the students every year. This is becoming unproductive particularly when students do not attend the institutions regularly but they enrol themselves only for getting scholarship amount. The state government is also taking active initiative for the implementation of Sarva Shiksha Abhiyan. The Programe seeks functional decentralisation right down to the school level in order to improve community participation. Involvement of the

Panchayati Raj Institutions/Tribal Councils, NGOs, teachers, activists and women's organizations would strengthen the accountability in implementation of the various programmes. The policy for universalisation of elementary eduction has to focus on a universal access and enrolment, universal retention of children up to 14 years of age, and policy framework for bringing about substantial improvement in the quality of education including — improvement in educational infrastructure, standardization and regular review of curricula, improvement in teaching aids, practices and training — to enable children to achieve essential levels of learning. To the extent that the legislative support helps in bringing these elements of the educational strategy into a sharper public focus, the initiation of the process for enactment of a central law making elementary education compulsory is a step in the right direction. This could increase school enrolments and retention over successive classes by acting as a deterrent to parents from premature withdrawal of their children from schools, as well as motivate the social interest groups and administrative machinery to encourage children to attend schools. Above all, the legislation is seen as an enabling framework for bringing about attitudinal changes - the attitude of parents towards their children's education, the state attitude towards children and towards improving the quality of educational system. (NHDR : 2001).

In short, human resources in any region have three aspects increasingly more important in the sequel: (1) physical fitness - relating to physical effort, easily captured by the number of workers, their general health (corporal), number of man-hours devoted to work, etc, (2) dexterity - agility, skill, expertise, ability, proficiency - inculcated by training, and (3) attitude, outlook, mindset - imbibed modernization ideals (in the sense of Gunnar Myrdal,) and their practice at mass level. This third aspect makes *'soft resources'* or the social capital.' The first two aspects of human resources are generally considered in planning for development. However, there is a need to devise suitable and practical programmes for preserving and generating social capital. It is a difficult area often bypassed by the economic planners under the umbrella of non-economic factors. But this neglect is counter-productive. We should note what Myrdal once said - there are no economic problems, social problems, political 'problems and so on. There are problems, and their economic, social and political aspects.

REFERENCES

HDRC, www,undp,ocg

Mishra, SK: Issues and Problems in Human Resource Development in NER. http//www.freewebs.com/nehu in economics/hrdner.pdf

National Human Development Report 2001 (NHDR)

Provisional Population. Totals ,Chapter 7,Census of India 2001 ,Series 1, India, Paper 1 of 2001

Table 6.6
Human Development Index for the States of NEI-1981

States/UTs	Rural		Urban		Combined		Gender Disparity Index	
	Value	Rank	Value	Rank	Value	Rank	Value	Rank
Arunachal Pradesh	0.228	28	0.419	24	0.242	31	0.537	28
Assan	0.261	26	0.380	28	0.272	26	0.462	32
Manipur	0.440	02	0.553	05	0.461	04	0.802	03
Meghalaya	0.293	20	0.442	21	0.317	21	0.799	12
Mizorum	0.381	09	0.558	04	0.411	08	0.502	18
Nagaland	0.295	19	0.519	08	0.328	20	0.783	16
Tripura	0.264	23	0.498	12	0.287	24	0.422	31
All-India	0.263		0.442		0.302		0.620	

Source : National Human Development Report-2001

Table 6.7
Rural Literacy Rate in NE States-(1981-2001)

(Percentage)

States/UTs	1981			1991			2001		
	Male	Female	Persons	Male	Female	Persons	Male	Female	Persons
Arunachal Pradesh	32.12	11.89	22.81	47.00	25.31	37.02	58.09	37.56	48.34
Assam	-	-	-	58.66	39.19	49.32	69.02	52.25	60.92
Manipur	59.66	30.03	45.09	67.64	43.26	55.79	74.50	55.88	65.33
Meghalaya	38.59	30.00	34.39	44.83	37.12	41.05	59.90	54.02	57.00
Mizorum	74.89	62.92	69.17	77.36	67.03	72.47	84.38	76.17	80.46
Nagaland	54.15	35.95	45.62	63.42	50.36	57.23	67.73	57.87	62.99
Tripura	57.76	33.02	45.78	67.07	44.33	56.08	78.89	61.05	70.23
All-India	49.59	21.70	36.01	57.87	30.62	44.69	71.18	46.58	59.21

Source : National Human Development Report-2001

Note : 1. Census not held in Assam in 1981.

2. Literacy Rate is defined as the proportion of literates to the population in the age group 7+.

3. For Census 1981, Literacy rate was defined for the population 6+. To ensure comparability in this exercise it has been estimated for the population 7+.

Table 6.8
Urban Literacy Rate in NE States-(1981-2001)

(Percentage)

States/UTs	1981			1991			2001		
	Male	Female	Persons	Male	Female	Persons	Male	Female	Persons
Arunachal Pradesh	70.42	51.94	63.75	77.99	62.23	71.59	85.61	70.60	78.82
Assam	-	-	-	84.37	73.32	79.39	89.88	81.03	85.76
Manipur	76.73	47.66	62.44	82.11	58.67	70.53	88.72	71.47	80.04
Meghalaya	80.17	69.36	75.09	85.72	77.32	81.74	89.90	84.30	87.12
Mizorum	92.44	86.04	89.46	95.15	91.65	93.45	96.97	95.69	96.35
Nagaland	79.88	70.18	76.12	85.94	79.10	83.10	89.01	82.09	85.95
Tripura	90.34	76.02	86.36	89.00	76.93	83.09	93.51	85.36	89.51
All-India	-	-	-	-	-	-	86.42	72.94	80.06

Source : National Human Development Report-2001

Note :
1. Census not held in Assam in 1981.
2. Literacy Rate is defined as the proportion of literates to the population in the age group 7+.
3. For Census 1981, Literacy rate was defined for the population 6+. To ensure comparability in this exercise it has been estimated for the population 7+.

Table 6.9
Literacy Rate of Scheduled Tribes in NE States-(1981-1991)

(Percentage)

States/UTs	1981			1991		
	Male	Female	Persons	Male	Female	Persons
Arunachal Pradesh	20.79	7.31	14.04	44.00	24.94	34.45
Assam	-	-	-	58.93	38.98	49.16
Manipur	48.88	30.55	39.74	62.39	44.48	53.63
Meghalaya	34.19	28.91	31.55	49.78	43.63	46.71
Mizorum	64.12	55.12	59.63	86.66	78.70	82.73
Nagaland	47.32	32.99	40.32	66.27	54.51	60.59
Tripura	33.46	12.37	23.07	52.88	27.34	40.37
All-India	24.52	8.04	16.35	40.65	18.10	29.60

Source : National Human Development Report-2001

Note :
1. Census not held in Assam in 1981.
2. Literacy Rate is defined as the proportion of literates to the population in the age group 7+.
3. For Census 1981, Literacy rate was defined for the population 6+. To ensure comparability in this exercise it has been reestimated for the population 7+.

Table 6.10
Literates/Illiterates in the age group 7-14 years in NE States-(1981-1991)

(Percentage)

States/UTs	Boys				Girls				Children			
	Litrates		Illiterates		Literates		illiterates		Literates		Illiterates1	
	1981	1991	1981	1991	1981	1991	1981	1991	1981	1991	1981	1991
Arunachal Pradesh	38.89	60.84	61.11	39.16	23.06	47.60	76.94	52.40	31.31	54.47	68.69	45.53
Assam	-	66.77	-	33.23	-	58.17	-	41.83	-	62.55	-	37.45
Manipur	63.79	75.50	36.21	24.80	50.94	67.29	49.06	32.71	57.46	71.19	42.54	28.71
Meghalaya	41.26	50.29	58.74	49.71	42.78	51.11	57.22	48.89	42.01	50.70	57.99	49.30
Mizorum	69.79	85.01	30.21	14.99	62.90	82.10	30.80	17.90	69.50	83.55	30.50	16.45
Nagaland	57.38	71.01	42.62	28.99	50.34	66.90	49.66	33.10	53.96	69.01	46.04	30.99
Tripura	60.36	74.41	39.64	25.59	50.02	66.38	49.98	33.62	16.44	70.47	83.56	29.53
All-India	60.58	71.44	39.42	28.56	41.57	56.23	58.43	43.77	51.49	64.16	48.51	35.84

Source: National Human Development Report-2001

Table 6.11
Adult Literacy Rate-(combined) in NE States-(1981-1991)

(Percentage)

States/UTs	1981			1991		
	Male	Female	Persons	Male	Female	Persons
Arunachal Pradesh	34.02	11.01	23.77	48.69	23.59	37.53
Assam	-	-	-	60.25	37.63	49.58
Manipur	64.27	29.19	47.04	70.62	41.86	56.63
Meghalaya	48.61	35.04	42.06	54.08	42.61	48.55
Mizorum	82.22	68.41	75.77	85.79	77.39	81.86
Nagaland	58.92	37.06	49.14	66.59	50.58	59.28
Tripura	61.89	33.57	48.25	69.34	44.06	57.15
All-India	54.92	25.72	40.83	61.89	34.09	48.54

Source : National Human Development Report-2001

Note: 1. Census not held in Assam in 1981 and Jammu & Kashmir in 1991.

2. Adult Literacy rate is percentage of literates in age-group 15 years and above to population in that age group.

Table 6.12
Adult Literacy Rate-(Rural) in NE States-(1981-1991)

(Percentage)

States/UTs	1981			1991		
	Male	Female	Persons	Male	Female	Persons
Arunachal Pradesh	30.75	8.93	20.84	43.80	19.13	32.61
Assam	-	-	-	56.61	33.23	45.47
Manipur	59.98	25.05	42.82	66.50	37.43	52.40
Meghalaya	40.46	27.86	34.30	45.68	34.64	40.30
Mizorum	8.20	62.81	70.94	77.51	65.01	71.71
Nagaland	54.42	32.80	44.41	62.08	46.05	54.55
Tripura	57.91	27.99	43.50	65.31	37.63	51.99
All-India	47.39	17.60	32.79	54.89	24.92	40.34

Source : National Human Development Report-2001

Note: 1. Census not held in Assam in 1981 and Jammu & Kashmir in 1991.

2. Adult Literacy rate is percentage of literates in age-group 15 years and above to population in that age group.

Table 6.13
Adult Literacy Rate-(Urban) in NE States-(1981-1991)

(Percentage)

States/UTs	1981			1991		
	Male	Female	Persons	Male	Female	Persons
Arunachal Pradesh	69.61	48.66	62.63	77.07	57.64	69.55
Assam	-	-	-	83.77	70.66	78.00
Manipur	76.15	40.67	58.72	81.38	53.16	67.53
Meghalaya	80.02	66.28	73.72	85.21	75.01	80.47
Mizorum	93.47	85.24	89.74	95.10	90.83	93.08
Nagaland	79.83	67.38	75.34	85.40	76.45	81.88
Tripura	90.81	73.59	82.47	89.03	74.76	82.08
All-India	76.29	51.90	65.11	80.14	59.86	70.68

Source : National Human Development Report-2001

Note : 1. Census not held in Assam in 1981 and Jammu & Kashmir in 1991.

2. Adult Literacy rate is percentage of literates in age-group 15 years and above to population in that age group.

Table 6.14
Age-specific Enrolment Ratias-Rural in NE States

(Percentage)

States/UTs	Age Group 6 to below 11 years						Age group 11 to below 14 years					
	1981			1991			1981			1991		
	Boys	Girls	Children	Boys	Girls	Children	Boys	Girls	Children	Boys	Girls	Children
Arunachal Pradesh	37.4	22.1	30.0	39.8	30.3	35.2	52.7	28.0	40.9	66.3	50.3	58.6
Assam	-	-	-	47.0	40.8	43.9	-	-	-	66.0	56.1	61.2
Manipur	49.6	40.0	44.9	47.0	42.1	44.6	71.9	52.3	62.2	73.3	64.4	68.9
Meghalaya	30.0	30.8	30.4	27.6	27.9	27.8	41.0	43.2	42.1	47.1	49.3	48.2
Mizorum	67.7	67.0	67.4	53.1	50.4	51.8	80.6	72.8	76.8	71.9	66.1	69.0
Nagaland	46.9	41.0	44.0	45.5	41.9	43.7	70.7	60.7	65.8	69.2	65.2	67.2
Tripura	54.6	46.4	50.6	53.2	47.3	50.3	65.6	49.8	57.8	76.1	65.4	70.9
All-India	50.6	31.4	41.3	52.3	39.3	46.0	57.6	28.1	43.7	67.6	44.4	56.7

Source : National Human Developmet Report - 2001
Note : Age-Specific Enrolment Ratio = (Estimated enrolment in an age group/Estimated child population in that age group) × 100

Table 6.15
Age-Specific Enrolment Ratios in NE States —(Urban)

(Percentage)

States/UTs	Age Group 6 to below 11 years						Age group 11 to below 14 years					
	1981			1991			1981			1991		
	Boys	Girls	Children	Boys	Girls	Children	Boys	Girls	Children	Boys	Girls	Children
Arunachal Pradesh	70.4	59.1	65.0	63.3	57.6	60.6	77.2	64.7	71.6	83.0	75.1	79.3
Assam	-	-	-	69.6	66.0	67.8	-	-	-	83.8	78.8	81.3
Manipur	70.7	64.0	67.4	59.0	56.4	57.7	88.5	75.9	82.3	82.1	77.1	79.6
Meghalaya	79.1	76.8	77.9	72.9	70.2	71.5	84.6	81.1	82.8	86.7	83.5	85.1
Mizorum	90.4	90.1	90.2	78.9	78.5	78.7	94.0	91.7	92.8	89.3	86.8	88.0
Nagaland	80.9	77.3	79.2	66.5	64.4	65.5	85.5	82.2	83.9	84.5	82.9	83.7
Tripura	82.7	78.4	80.6	69.7	66.7	68.2	89.1	82.8	85.9	89.2	85.1	87.1
All-India	72.8	64.9	69.0	70.7	65.8	68.3	76.6	64.5	70.8	81.0	73.6	77.5

Source: National Human Development Report-2001.

Note: Age-Specific Enrolment Ratio = (Estimated enrolment in an age group/Estimated child population in that age group) × 100

Table 6.16
Girls Enrolled in Various School Stages in NE States, 1978—Combined

(Percentage)

States/UTs	I-V			VI-VIII			IX onwards		
	All	SC	ST	All	SC	ST	All	SC	ST
Arunachal Pradesh	32.09	29.50	31.12	29.01	29.16	26.07	23.65	37.50	19.48
Assam	42.13	40.84	41.52	38.97	37.07	35.81	35.73	34.15	31.34
Manipur	44.27	48.68	44.66	38.93	44.06	38.40	35.28	39.26	31.64
Meghalaya	49.33	47.65	49.71	45.68	39.89	46.56	43.15	22.84	44.38
Mizorum	48.12	-	48.12	45.96	-	45.92	44.00	-	43.89
Nagaland	44.34	-	44.65	42.24	-	42.15	36.64	-	37.61
Tripura	41.60	40.73	32.11	40.27	34.55	28.79	39.62	27.21	27.24
All-India	38.27	34.36	33.29	32.0	25.82	26.97	28.69	21.53	26.70

Source : National Human Development Report-2001

Table 6.17
Girls Enrolled in Various School Stages in NE States, 1993—Combined

(Percentage)

States/UTs	I-V			VI-VIII			IX-X			XI-XII		
	All	SC	ST	All	SC	ST	All	SC	ST	All	SC	ST
Arunachal Pradesh	43.28	39.80	44.26	40.53	37.15	40.90	37.13	41.30	36.50	30.25	35.00	26.21
Assam	45.46	44.97	47.03	44.81	44.65	44.55	44.99	45.13	44.26	36.97	35.80	37.33
Manipur	46.91	47.64	45.55	46.49	42.61	44.79	46.66	42.47	43.34	35.88	17.43	40.43
Meghalaya	50.14	47.30	50.46	48.56	40.94	49.62	46.88	43.20	48.38	41.87	43.33	55.80
Mizorum	47.36	51.42	47.39	48.30	36.00	48.39	49.97	23.81	50.05	-	-	-
Nagaland	47.90	44.31	48.02	49.11	44.53	49.24	46.26	43.15	46.24	38.33	-	38.33
Tripura	45.75	46.21	43.45	44.63	43.18	40.90	43.06	40.45	37.31	36.19	32.33	26.06
All-India	43.16	41.66	41.45	39.62	36.25	35.77	36.47	32.31	32.10	35.93	30.29	27.62

Source : National Human Development Report - 2001

Table 6.18
Drop-out Rates in Classes I-V in NE States

(Percentage)

States/UTs	1981-82			1992-93			1998-99(Provisional)		
	Boys	Girls	Children	Boys	Girls	Children	Boys	Girls	Children
Arunachal Pradesh	74.6	72.2	73.9	58.72	63.02	60.54	48.28	45.10	46.89
Assam	59.4	66.6	62.5	51.66	59.93	55.37	40.87	42.43	41.56
Manipur	80.1	82.3	81.1	66.94	67.60	67.25	51.42	53.9	52.59
Meghalaya	75.1	76.8	76.0	12.92	13.92	13.39	61.07	63.77	62.44
Mizorum#	65.2	69.7	67.3	57.1	59.52	58.24	51.60	52.08	51.82
Nagaland	71.1	71.5	71.3	34.68	36.52	35.59	36.71	35.09	35.94
Tripura#	55.9	55.4	55.7	59.06	60.46	59.70	50.28	53.91	51.95
All-India	51.1	57.3	53.5	48.83	46.67	45.01	38.23	41.34	39.58

Source : National Human Development Report - 2001
Notes 1 # Figures relate to 1997-98 taken from VI All India Educational Survey.

Table 6.19
Drop-out Rates in Classes I-VIII in NE States

(Percentage)

States/UTs	1981-82			1992-93			1998-99(Provisional)		
	Boys	Girls	Children	Boys	Girls	Children	Boys	Girls	Children
Arunachal Pradesh	84.40	83.60	84.20	72.55	71.01	71.93	67.67	65.86	66.78
Assam	81.80	84.20	82.50	68.35	70.36	69.22	68.26	72.31	70.08
Manipur	85.10	88.20	86.40	67.75	67.80	67.77	45.36	47.02	46.15
Meghalaya	88.50	88.50	88.50	50.63	49.90	50.29	77.71	78.11	77.91
Mizorum	78.00	80.60	79.30	66.64	62.05	64.37	68.50	65.75	67.20
Nagaland	86.80	89.20	87.80	36.24	37.37	37.45	46.46	38.95	42.98
Tripura	71.20	74.50	74.40	68.85	70.06	69.39	69.58	71.06	70.26
All-India	68.50	77.70	72.10	58.23	65.21	61.10	54.40	60.09	56.82

Source : National Human Development Report-2001

Table 6.20
Intensity of formal Education in NE States - 1978

(Years)

States/UTs	Rural			Urban			Combined		
	Boys	Girls	Children	Boys	Girls	Children	Boys	Girls	Children
Arunachal Pradesh	2.82	2.65	2.77	4.94	4.25	4.70	3.01	2.81	2.95
Assam	3.70	3.40	3.58	5.32	5.01	5.19	3.91	3.64	3.80
Manipur	3.67	3.16	3.46	5.62	5.15	5.41	4.08	3.63	3.89
Meghalaya	2.99	2.81	2.90	5.09	5.03	5.06	3.31	3.15	3.23
Mizorum	3.94	3.74	3.84	4.74	4.72	4.73	4.08	3.93	4.01
Nagaland	3.61	3.39	3.51	5.40	5.15	5.29	3.81	3.59	3.71
Tripura	3.56	3.36	3.48	5.84	5.69	5.77	3.94	3.87	3.91
All-India	3.83	3.27	3.64	5.16	4.69	4.97	4.19	3.76	4.03

Source : National Human Development Report-2001

Note : Intensity of formal education has been estimated as the weighted average of the enrolled students from Class I to Class XII (where weights being 1 for Class 1, 2 for Class II and so on) to the total enrolment in Classes I to Class XII.

Table 6.21
Accessibility to Schools in Rural Areas in NE States - 1978

(Percentage)

States/UTs	Population with primary schools			Population with upper primary schools		
	Within habitation	Up to 0.5 km#	Total up to 0.5 km	Within habitation	Up to 1.0 km#	Total up to 1.0 km
Arunachal Pradesh	55.90	1.72	57.62	18.14	3.75	21.89
Assam	81.34	6.12	87.46	20.91	14.66	35.57
Manipur	92.82	2.39	95.21	38.62	16.71	55.33
Meghalaya	76.12	7.38	83.50	15.72	13.58	29.30
Mizorum	74.54	-	74.54	64.32	0.66	64.98
Nagaland	98.35	0.61	98.96	50.72	6.25	56.97
Tripura	54.42	10.48	64.90	19.79	18.74	38.53
All-India	78.53	6.60	85.13	33.47	13.10	46.57

Source : National Human Development Report - 2001

Note :
1. # But not within the habitation.
2. Primary Stage refers to Class I to V and Upper Primary to Class VI to VIII.
3. Accessibility to Schools is defined as percentage of population having access to a school within the indicated distance.

Table 6. 22
Accessibility to Schools in Rural Areas in NE States — 1993

(Percentage)

States/UTs	Population with primary schools			Population with upper primary schools		
	Within habitation	Up to 0.5 km#	Total up to 0.5 km	Within habitation	Up to 1.0 km#	Total up to 1.0 km
Arunachal Pradesh	70.12	3.78	73.90	33.13	6.80	39.93
Assam	66.27	13.93	80.20	22.40	26.69	49.09
Manipur	82.26	7.81	90.07	37.25	25.60	62.85
Meghalaya	74.05	6.70	80.75	25.57	21.21	46.78
Mizorum	94.30	1.10	95.40	77.58	3.00	80.58
Nagaland	92.36	1.32	93.68	47.76	15.32	63.08
Tripura	55.43	13.13	68.56	24.92	28.38	53.30
All-India	77.81	7.69	85.50	37.02	19.89	56.91

Source: National Human Development Report-2001

Note : 1. # But not within the habitation.
2. Primary Stage refers to Class I to V and Upper Primary to Class VI to VIII.
3. Accessibility to Schools is defined as percentage of population having access to a school within the indicated distance.

Table 6.23
Teacher-Pupil Ratio in NE States

(Percentage)

States/UTs	1982-83			1992-93			1997-98		
	Primary	Upper primary	Secon-dary	Primary	Upper primary	Secon-dary	Primary	Upper primary	Secon-dary
Arunachal Pradesh	33	21	21	32	23	14	36	27	29
Assam	35	24	25	39	31	28	37	24	21
Manipur	18	21	20	18	11	17	19	19	21
Meghalaya	31	17	22	36	19	24	40	17	19
Mizorum	29	15	13	30	12	11	28	10	9
Nagaland	21	15	23	19	21	27	21	19	25
Tripura	41	29	24	23	25	23	18	15	17
All-India	40	34	29	45	43	29	42	37	29

Source : National Human Development Report-2001

Table 6.24
Number of Schools per Thousand Population in NE States

States/UTs	1982-83		1992-93		1997-98	
	Primary	Upper primary	Primary	Upper primary	Primary	Upper primary
Arunachal Pradesh	12.39	3.29	10.53	4.52	8.21	4.64
Assam	7.71	3.22	8.89	3.07	8.62	3.58
Manipur	14.62	4.29	13.10	5.17	8.69	4.02
Meghalaya	22.87	5.32	17.97	5.30	13.38	6.05
Mizorum	-	-	12.65	10.68	11.17	11.1
Nagaland	13.71	6.34	8.89	4.08	6.80	4.56
Tripura	6.71	1.77	6.81	2.58	4.14	1.77
All-India	5.70	2.44	5.75	2.69	5.04	2.75

Source : National Human Development Report - 2001

Note : For Mizorum population for the age group 6-11 and 11-14 was not available for 1982-83 and 1992-93.

Table 6.25
Composition of Public Spending in NE States — Some Critical Ratios — 1980 -81

(Percentage)

States/UTs	Public Expn. Ratio	Development Expn. Ratio	Social sector Expn. Ratio	Education Expn. Ratio	Health Expn. Ratio	Amenities Expn. Ratio	Other social Expn. Ratio
Arunachal Pradesh	-	-	-	-	-	-	-
Assam	30.13	51.43	22.45	12.76	5.23	1.03	3.43
Manipur	72.90	53.29	25.06	12.25	8.66	0.72	3.44
Meghalaya	50.85	63.59	29.73	9.97	15.34	2.09	2.33
Mizorum	-	-	-	-	-	-	-
Nagaland	138.19	50.93	22.88	8.03	9.57	2.20	3.08
Tripura	49.98	65.50	31.39	11.60	4.57	1.3	14.19
Central govt.	14.80	54.70	5.30	2.70	1.40	0.40	0.80
All-India	-	70.42	29.12	13.89	7.10	1.14	7.00

Source : National Human Development Report - 2001

Note :
1. Public Expenditure in this table includes debt service and repayments of loans of the State Governments.
2. Public Expenditure Ratio is total public expenditure as a proportion of Gross States Domestic Product.
3. Total development expenditure (including social services and economic services); Social Sector expenditure, including expenditure on education, health, amenities (i.e. water supply & sensation, housing and urban development) and other Social services (incluidng welfare of SC, ST & OBC; social security and welfare etc.) have been expressed as a ratio of total public expenditure.
4. For the Central Government, the ratio have been expressed as proportion of GDP and Central Government Expenditure net of loans and advances to States.

Table 6.26
Composition of Public Spending in NE States—Some Critical Ratios — 1990-91

(Percentage)

States/UTs	Public Expn. Ratio	Development Expn. Ratio	Social sector Expn. Ratio	Education Expn. Ratio	Health Expn. Ratio	Amenities Expn. Ratio	Other social Expn. Ratio
Arunachal Pradesh	78.30	75.72	25.18	13.31	4.51	5.77	1.60
Assam	25.32	64.75	30.80	16.94	5.04	4.74	4.08
Manipur	55.17	73.58	31.82	17.68	4.40	5.91	3.83
Meghalaya	45.58	74.70	34.71	15.63	6.18	10.43	2.47
Mizorum	147.26	55.80	23.23	9.47	3.39	6.87	3.50
Nagaland	84.30	66.40	28.33	10.15	6.30	8.97	2.91
Tripura	59.43	72.81	37.91	17.62	5.91	4.34	10.04
Central govt.	17.70	48.10	6.40	3.50	1.50	0.40	1.00
All-India		69.57	32.89	17.36	5.88	3.86	5.79

Source : National Human Development Report - 2001

Note :
1. Public Expenditure in this table includes debt service and repayments of loans of the State Governments.
2. Public Expenditure Ratio is total public expenditure as a proportion of Gross States Domestic Product.
3. Total development expenditure (including social services and economic services); Social Sector expenditure, including expenditure on education, health, amenities (i.e. water supply & sensation, housing and urban development) and other Social services (incluidng welfare of SC, ST & OBC; social security and welfare etc.) have been expressed as a ratio of total public expenditure.
4. For the Central Government, the ratio have been expressed as proportion of GDP and Central Government Expenditure net of loans and advances to States.

Table 6.27
Composition of Public Spending in NE States—Same Critical Ratios — 1998-99

(Percentage)

States/UTs	Public Expn. Ratio	Development Expn. Ratio	Social sector Expn. Ratio	Education Expn. Ratio	Health Expn. Ratio	Amenities Expn. Ratio	Other social Expn. Ratio
Arunachal Pradesh	65.09	72.98	26.27	12.04	5.43	6.42	2.38
Assam	20.50	62.39	39.07	26.34	4.65	3.30	4.49
Manipur	42.84	63.37	32.95	18.52	4.67	4.88	4.89
Meghalaya	33.63	69.10	35.19	16.95	7.22	8.64	2.38
Mizorum	-	71.16	35.35	12.97	4.93	11.58	5.87
Nagaland	-53.89	-2534	-9.55	-5.39	-7.37	-3.03	
Tripura	44.52	62.50	35.96	17.23	4.69	7.09	6.95
Central govt.	13.70	34.0	-8.20	3.90	1.80	1.00	1.40
All-India	-	61.76	33.07	17.39	5.78	4.53	5.38

Source : National Human Development Report - 2001

Note :
1. Public Expenditure in this table includes debt service and repayments of loans of the State Governments.
2. Public Expenditure Ratio is total public expenditure as a proportion of Gross States Domestic Product.
3. Total development expenditure (including social services and economic services); Social Sector expenditure, including expenditure on education, health, amenities (i.e. water supply & sensation, housing and urban development) and other Social services (incluidng welfare of SC, ST & OBC; social security and welfare etc.) have been expressed as a ratio of total public expenditure.
4. For the Central Government, the ratio have been expressed as proportion of GDP and Central Government Expenditure net of loans and advances to States.

Table 6.28
Public Spending on Education in NE States

(As a percentage of Gross State Domestic Product)

	1980-81	1990-91	1998-99
Arunachal Pradesh	78.30	75.72	25.18
Assam	25.32	64.75	30.80
Manipur	55.17	73.58	31.82
Meghalaya	45.58	74.70	34.71
Mizorum	147.26	55.80	23.23
Nagaland	84.30	66.40	28.33
Tripura	59.43	72.81	37.91
Central govt.	17.70	48.10	6.40
All-India	-	69.57	32.89

Source NHRD-2001

Note :
1. Public spending on education includes both revenue and capital expenditure for both plan and non-plan. It has been expressed as a ratio of Gross State Domestic Product.
2. Ratio are a moving average of two years, i.e. 1980-81 is average for the years 1980-81 and 1981-82.
3. For the Central Government the ratio shave been expressed as proportion of GDP,
4. The Central Government figures for 1998-99 is a moving average of the period 1996-98.

7

IMPACT OF EDUCATIONAL ATTAINMENT ON FERTILITY :
A CASE STUDY OF TRIPURA

– Anil Kumar Das

Fertility of women is a bilogical phenomenon. Several factors viz, economic, social, cultural and others affect the levels and differentials of fertility among different population groups or among different sub-groups of the same population. Study of differential fertility is thus, very much important in identifying the factors responsible for high or low levels of fertility among various sub-groups.

Among the factors which directly or indirectly influence the fertility of women of any society, education, especially female education, is perhaps one of the most important factor. Usually women are regarded as conservative elements and habituated to stay behind the screen. In spite of equal opportunities for both men and women, it has been observed that the performance of women is slower than men. Because women are tied by various traditional, social and cultural rules and regulations. For beinging socio-cultural change, women's education is considered an important factor (Jena : 1994). Again, in overall development process, education is regarded as the most essential. So, education is used as an important powerful instrument for socio-economic upliftment (Sinha, 1996). The increased education of women in particular, frequently plays an important role in changing attitude among women to their traditional role as homemaker and bearer of children.

David Madelbaum (1974) has observed that the joint family system, religion and urbanization are not the critical variables affecting child bearing behaviour. According to him, the significant factors tending to lower birth rates are higher education and greater affluence, which are both goals and symptoms of development. In another study, it is observed that education influences fertility directly by altering the attitudes and behavioural patterns of individuals, and indirectly by affecting such factors as age at marriage and jointly by operating with other aspects of modernization such as urbanization and industrialization (Holsinger & Kasarda: 1976). Phillips Cutright (1983) observed that literacy levels are more closely related to fertility change than the macro economic factors like urbanization, income, energy consumption or percentage of the labour force engaged in agriculture. Besides these, numerous studies have showed that education is highly negatively correlated with decreased fertility (Martin Teresa Castro: 1995; Rindfuss Ronald R et all: 1996; De wit Margaret L and Fernando Rajulton, 1992; Dodoo F. Nii-Amoo: 1992; Jain Anrudh K: 1985; Bloom, David E and James Trussell: 1984). Increased education leads to lower fertility for three principal reasons. Women with higher levels of education delay childbearing, desire fewer children and more often use effective methods of modern birth control (Castro: 95; Jain: 1985). Women who have their first child at a later age have fewer remaining reproductive years, thus they have fewer children. A study of United States fertility patterns found that most high school graduates have their first child between the ages of 21 and 23 while college graduates delay child bearing until 27 to 29 years (Rindfuss: 1989). A negative association between the education of women and fertility was observed by J. R. Rele and Tara Kanitkar (1974). Similarly, an inverse relation between education of couples and fertility among Meiteis in Manipur was also observed (Choudhury and Devi:1997). They also observed that Muslim couples in Manipur however do not show any such clear cut relationship. When the education of husbands and wives are considered separately, it is found that education of Muslim women has very little effect on their fertility. The fertility of the women is, however, found to decrease with the increase of the educational status of the husbands. A study conducted on Jenu Karuba and Kadu Karuba tribes of Karnataka showed that education has not shown any significant reduction in fertility (Mutharayappa: 1994). Dandekar and Dandekar (1953) also could not find any consistent relationship between fertility and variation in the level of literacy in Pune. Again husband's education was found equally strongly related to wife's fertility when the other socio economic factors including wife's schooling were controlled, indicating that the schooling of both husband and wife contribute to lower fertility (UN: 1986). NFHS, India, 1992-93 (IIPS: 1995) also confirmed that differentials by education are substantial with current fertility - TFR declining steadily from 4 children per woman for illiterate women to 2.2 children per woman for women with at least a high school education. Fertility measured by mean number of 'children ever born[1] to women aged 40-49 year, is also higher among illiterate women than among women with at least a high school education. Deka (2003) also found that with the improvement in educational attainment the mean size of 'children ever born' decreases. In another study on Saharia, a primitive tribe of Madhya Pradesh, it is observed that the educational characteristic of husbands appears to influence fertility as the mean number of 'children ever born' is less i.e. 2.96 at aggregate level when they are literate and more and 3.76 when they are illiterate. In addition, mean number of 'children ever born' is lower when husbands are more educated (Biswas & Kapoor: 2003).

Materials and Methods

The present chapter is an attempt to focus the differential fertility of rural women of Tripura with the help of the explanatory variable educational attainment. To be specific, the study aims to examine the relationship between (a) fertility and woman's educational attainment[2] and (b) fertility and husband's educational attainment, with reference to rural women of Tripura.

The data for the present study have been collected from randomly selected 1200 households from the rural areas of Tripura by multistage stratified random sampling method. From the selected households 1350 'currently married women'[3] under reproductive span of life were studied. The fertility data were collected using scheduled questionnaire method. In the discourse, fertility has been considered as 'cohort fertility' measured by mean children ever born.[4]

To examine the levels and differentials fertility of currently married women of rural Tripura by educational attainment, the explanatory variable education is categorized into three groups viz. 'Illiterate', up to Primary level and above Primary level. The total surveyed population of currently married women, for the sake of simplicity henceforth be referred as 'women,' are classified again by 5-year age interval viz. 15-19, 20-24, 25-29, 30-34, 35-39, 40-44, and 45-49.

Result and Discussion

Table-7.1 depicts the mean number of children ever born per woman by present age and her educational attainment. From table 7.1 it is observed that the cohort fertility measured by mean children ever born for illiterate women increases with the increase of woman's age. Similar results are also found for women with educational level up to primary and above primary. For illiterate group the cohort fertility lies between 0.54 to 5.35 children per woman. For women with educational level up to primary, it is between 0.60 and 4.09. The fertility levels extend from 0.39 to 4.10 for those women who belong to above primary group. Almost for all age group the fertility decreases steadily with the increase of educational attainment of the women. Again, the fertility levels of illiterate, up to primary and above primary groups are 3.48, 2.79 and 2.04 children per woman respectively. It indicates that the illiterate women have more than one child than the women with educational level above primary. Thus, the fertility of women aged 15-49 year decreases with the improvement of the educational attainment in rural Tripura. The standardized averages of the respective groups also confirm this fact.

Table 7.1
Average number of children ever born per woman by age and by her educational attainment in Tripura

Age of woman	Educational Attainment of the woman		
	Illiterate	Up to Primary	Above Primary
15 - 19	0.54	0.60	0.39
20 - 24	1.58	1.58	1.02
25 - 29	2.66	2.62	1.79
30 - 34	3.94	3.23	2.67
35 -39	4.10	3.80	3.00
40 - 44	5.07	4.31	3.78
45 - 49	5.35	4.09	4.10
Average Number of Children ever born	3.48	2.79	2.04
Standardized Average	3.25	2.92	2.28

Source : Field Survey, 1996 - 97.

Population of Tripura may broadly be grouped as tribal and non-tribal. One third of the state's population is scheduled tribe and the rest is non-tribal. Nearly 83 percent of state's population lives in rural areas. Thus, the educational attainmnet and the fertility levels of tribes and non-tribes of rural Tripura have also been examined.

Table 7.2 reveals the mean number of children ever born per non-tribal women by age and by her educational status.

From Table 7.2 it is observed that the cohort fertility for illiterate women increases with the increase of the age of the women. Similar findings are observed for women with educational level up to Primary and above Primary. For 'illiterate' class fertility lies between 0.42 and 6.17 children per woman. For 'up to Primary' and 'above Primary' fertility ranges from 0.67 to 4.5 and from 0.31 to 4.17 children per woman respectively. From table 7.2 it is clear that the fertility of almost all the age groups decreases steadily with the advancement of the educational status of the non-tribal women. Further, the fertility levels of the 'illiterate', 'up to Primary' and 'above Primary' are 3.48, 2.82 and 2.07 children per woman respectively. The standardized averages of the corresponding classes are 3.35, 2.91 and 2.28 respectively. The fertility levels and the standardized averages indicate that higher fertility is associated with lower level of education of the non-tribal women.

Table 7.2

Average number of children ever born per non-tribal woman by age and by her educational attainment in Tripura

Age of woman	Educational Attainment of the woman		
	Illiterate	Up to Primary	Above Primary
15 - 19	0.42	0.67	0.31
20 - 24	1.64	1.70	1.07
25 - 29	2.78	2.64	1.76
30 - 34	4.26	3.00	2.61
35 -39	3.94	3.81	3.13
40 - 44	4.93	4.18	3.71
45 - 49	6.17	4.50	4.17
Average Number of Children ever born	3.48	2.82	2.07
Standardized Average	3.35	2.91	2.28

Source : Field Survey, 1996 - 97.

Table 7.3 describes the average number of children ever born per tribal woman by age and her educational level. From table 7.3 it is observed that the cohort fertility of the tribal women with educational level 'illiterate' or 'up to Primary' or 'above Primary' shows an upward trend with the increase of the age of the women. Again, the fertility for almost all the age groups goes on decreasing with the increased educational attainment. From table 7.3 it is observed that the fertility levels of the women belong to 'illiterate' or 'up to Primary' or 'above Primary' is 3.49, 2.71 and 1.97 mean children per women. It suggests that the differential fertility of the tribal women by educational attainment is substantial. The cohort fertility declines consistently from 3.49 children per woman for illiterate to 1.97 children per woman for tribal women with educational level 'above Primary'. Standardized averages also follow the same path. Thus marital fertility and educational attainment as observed are inversely related in rural areas in Tripura.

Table 7.3
Average number of children ever born per tribal woman by age and by her educational attainment in Tripura

Age of woman	Educational Attainment of the woman		
	Illiterate	Up to Primary	Above Primary
15 - 19	1.00	0.50	0.50
20 - 24	1.52	1.23	1.93
25 - 29	2.55	2.58	1.85
30 - 34	3.60	3.80	2.87
35 -39	4.23	3.78	2.64
40 - 44	5.18	5.00	4.00
45 - 49	4.58	3.00	4.00
Average Number of Children ever born	3.49	2.71	1.97
Standardized Average	3.15	2.98	2.28

Source : Field Survey, 1996 - 97.

It perhaps requires no mention that like woman's educational attainment, the educational status of the husband also plays an important role in reducing fertility rate. Thus, the relationship between fertility and the educational status of husband is examined. The educational level of the husbands is classified into four categories - 'illiterate', 'Up to Primary level' 'Above Primary but below Secondary' (Madhyamik) level and 'Secondary level and above'. Under these four heads the wives of the husbands, i.e. women of the sample are classified by 5-year age interval. The cohort fertility for each age interval under the categories is determined separately.

Table-7.4 depicts the average number of children ever born per currently married women by age and by educational attainment of their spouses. From Table 7.4 it is observed that husband's educational status infleunces strongly in reducing marital fertility. In each age group, fertility declines almost consistently with the improvement of educational level of the husbands. The average number of children ever born per woman of the four categories describes that fertility starts decreasing with the initiation of the educative process and it moves on decreasing with the increase of the educational level of the husbands. The women of the illiterate spouses have considerably higher fertility (3.47 children per woman) as compared to the women whose spouses have received education at the level of secondary or beyond (2.12 children per woman). It indicates that women whose husbands have crossed the secondary level or studied beyond have on an average more than one child less than that of the women living with illiterate husbands.

Table 7.4

Average number of children ever born by age and by the educational attainment of her spouse.

	Educational Attainment of the woman			
Age of woman Secondary	**Illiterate**	**Up to Primary**	**Above Primary but below Secondary**	**and Above**
15 - 19	0.62	0.45	0.53	0.22
20 - 24	1.59	1.45	1.36	0.98
25 - 29	2.72	2.66	2.16	1.76
30 - 34	4.04	3.55	3.39	2.40
35 -39	3.97	4.29	3.98	3.02
40 - 44	5.02	5.32	4.30	3.60
45 - 49	5.24	5.10	4.00	4.33
Average Number of Children ever born	3.47	3.19	2.60	2.12
Standardized Average	3.26	3.18	2.81	2.20

Source : Field Survey, 1996 - 97.

Table 7.5 depicts the fertility of non-tribal women by age and by the educational attainment of their spouses. Table 7.5 describes that the fertility of the women of illiterate spouses increase with the increase of the age of the woman. Similar observations have been found for the women when the educational level of their spouses being either up to Primary or above Primary but below secondary or secondary and above. Table 7.5 also describes that for almost all age groups fertility declines consistently with the improvement of the educational attainment of the spouses of the non-tribal women under study. Again, the fertility of the women of the different classes namely illiterate, up to Primary, above Primary but below Secondary and Secondary and above stratified according to the educational levels of the spouses of the women is 3.52, 2.89, 2.59 and 2.07 children per woman respectively. The standardized averages of the corresponding classes are 3.39, 3.04, 2.76 and 2.11. The mean children ever born and the standardized averages indicate the existence of negative association between fertility of non-tribal women and the educational status of their spouses.

Table 7.5
Average number of children ever born by age and by the educational attainment of her spouse (non-tribal)

Age of woman Secondary	Educational Attainment of the woman			
	Illiterate	Up to Primary	Above Primary but below Secondary	and Above
15 - 19	0.40	0.50	0.40	0.20
20 - 24	1.56	1.42	1.48	1.04
25 - 29	2.84	2.61	2.23	1:66
30 - 34	4.27	3.50	3.25	2.30
35 -39	3.85	4.05	3.93	2.96
40 - 44	5.29	4.25	4.29	3.25
45 - 49	6.70	5.36	3.00	4.20
Average Number of Children ever born	3.52	2.89	2.59	2.07
Standardized Average	3.39	3.04	2.76	2.11

Source : Field Survey, 1996 - 97.

Table 7.6 describes the average number of children ever born per tribal woman by age and by the educational status of her spouse. From Table 7.6 it is observed that when the spouses are classified according to their educational level as illiterate, up to Primary, above Primary but below Secondary and Secondary and above then the fertility of the tribal women are 3.41, 3.69, 2.61 and 2.19 respectively. The standardized averages of the corresponding classes are 3.14, 3.33, 2.83 and 2.33 children per woman respectively. The fertility measured by mean children ever born and the standardized averages exhibit the decreasing trend in fertility levels when the educational attainment of the spouses is in transit from no education to secondary and above level of education.

Table 7.6
Average number of children ever born by age and by the educational attainment of her spouse (tribal)

	Educational Attainment of the woman			
Age of woman	**Illiterate**	**Up to**	**Above Primary**	
Secondary		**Primary**	**but below**	**and**
			Secondary	**Above**
15 - 19	1.33	-	0.67	0.25
20 - 24	1.63	1.55	1.09	0.90
25 - 29	2.60	2.73	2.00	1.90
30 - 34	3.73	3.63	3.63	2.59
35 -39	4.09	4.50	4.05	3.13
40 - 44	4.83	6.60	4.33	4.00
45 - 49	3.91	4.57	4.75	4.50
Average Number of Children ever born	3.41	3.69	2.61	2.19
Standardized Average	3.14	3.33	2.83	2.33

Source : Field Survey, 1996 - 97.

Conclusion

In conclusion, it may be emphasized here that the cutting point of women's educational attainment for exhibiting a negative relationship with fertility is the level of above primary. Women who either have passed the primary level or have studied beyond that level generally have on an average 1 to 1.5 children less than who are illiterate. It is observed that women with Madhyamik or H.S. or above educational attainment have less than the average of 'above primary group.' Further, for exhibiting a negative relationship between husband's educational status and fertility, the cutting point in husband's educational level is the level of secondary or above. The husbands who had either completed the Madhyamik examination (secondary level) or had studied beyond that level usually have on an average 1 to 1.5 children which is remarkably less as compared to illiterate ones. Thus if the proportion of educated couples in the society can be increased to a substantial extent, there would be decline in fertility rate. These findings have important implication for strategy of planning for the development of the state. Thus the value of the education, particularly women's education in the state may be emphasized to a great extent for future reduction of fertility rate.

NOTES

1. As per United Nations recommendations, 'number of children ever born' include all live born children whether legitimate or illegitimate or whether born of present or of the previous marriages or whether they are living or dead at the time of the survey or where they may living. (Principles and Recommendations for the 1970 population censuses, Statistical paper, series M. No. 44, United Nations).
2. Literacy is defined as the ability of a person to both read and write, with understanding, a short simple statement on his every day life (Principles and Recommendations for the 1970 population census, Statistical paper, Series M. No. 44, United Nations). A person who cannot meet this criterion is regarded as Illiterate.
3. 'Current married woman' means the married woman in the reproductive age 15-49 year living with her husband.

4. When one group of women with common characteristics (born in the same year or married in the same year) is traced throughout their reproductive life span, the performance each year is recorded, giving finally the total number of children born to the group. In this way the mean number of children ever born is obtained. (Pollard, A. H.; Yusuf, Farhat; Pollard, G. N. 'Demographic technique, Pergamon Press (1981). The fertility determined in this way is the cohort fertility.

REFERENCES

Biswas, R. K. and Kapoor, A. K. -"Education and its Effect on Fertility and Mortality Differentials Among a Primitive Tribe of Madhya Pradesh", Indian Journal of Population Education, 23 (2003).

Bloom, D.E. and Trussell,J - "What Are The Determinants of Delayed Child Bearing And Permanent Childlessness In The United States" Demography, 21(4): 591-611, (1984).

Castro, M.T.-"Women's Education And Fertility : Results From 26 Demographic Health Surveys" Studies in Family Planning, 26(4): 187-202, (1995).

Choudhury, B; Devi, M.- "Fertility differentials in Manipur : A Study on the Meiteis and the Muslims", J. Hum.Ecol., 8, (1997).

Cutright, Phillips 'The Ingredients of Recent Fertility Decline in Developing Countries', International Family Planning Perspectives, 9, (1983).

Dandekar, V.M. and Dandekar, K.- "Survey of Fertility and Mortality in Poona District", Publication 27, Gokhale Institute of Politics and Economics, Poona (1953).

Deka, N.K., 'Some Aspects of Fertility among Muslims of Barpeda District : An Empirical Study', Journal of North-East India Council for Social Science Research, 27, (2003).

De Wit, M. L. and Fernando, R.-"Education and timing of Parenthood Among Canadian Women: A cohort Analysis", Social Biology, Spring-Summer, 29(1-2): 109-122 (1992).

Dodoo, F. Nii-Amoo - "Female Education, Age, Parity and Reproduction Cessation in Ghana", Social Biology, Spring-Summer, 39(1-2): 102-108 (1992).

Holsinger, D.R. and Kasarda, J.-"Populaltion and Development - The Search for Selective Intervention", Ridker Ronald G (ed), John opkins University Press (1976).

Jain, A.K.-"The Impact of Development and Population policies on Fertility In India", Studies in Family Planning, 16(4): 181-198, (1985).

Jena, K. - "Progress of the Educated Tribal Women", Man in India, 74(1): 81-86, (1994).

Mandelbaum, D.G. - "Human Fertility in India", Berkeley, University of California Press (1974).

Mutharayappa, R. - "Factors Affecting Fertility Among Tribal", Man and Development, 16(4), 63-79, (1994).

IIPS, 'National Family Health Survey (MCH and Family Planning) India, 1992-93, Bombay, 1995.

Rele, J. R., Kanitkar, T. "Residence Background and Fertility in Greater Bombay", Population Studies, 28, (1974).

Rindfuss, Ronald R et al - "Education And the Changing Age Pattern of American Fertility : 1963-1989", Demography, 33(3), 277-290, (1996).

Sinha, R - "Equalization of Educational Opportunities - Scheduled Castes and Scheduled Tribes : Problems and Future Strategies", Man in India, 76(2), 141-159, (1996).

United Nations - "Education and Fertility : Selected Findings

8

LEVEL OF INCOME AND HUMAN DEVELOPMENT

A CASE OF THREE NORTH EASTERN STATES

– Anup Kumar Datta

Introduction

The Northeastern region of India consists of eight small states. Although being strategically significant, and having immense development potentials, the entire region has been subjected to utter underdevelopment and neglect. Acute poverty and unemployment happens to be the most burning issue, which needs to be addressed on war footing. The region is least known and least explored. The peculiar geographical location and severe communication gap have fuelled extremist movement. Industrialization in this region *is* not even in infant stage. The region hardly attracts private initiative for investment. Government initiative is the only hope for any positive change in the living condition of the people of this region. On this count, it would be worthwhile to review the achievement of the state in performing certain objectives essential for human development vis-a-vis growth in income.

Objective

This chapter is designed to focus issues related to the progress in the field of human development in three northeastern states viz. Assam, Meghalaya and Tripura. It seeks to investigate the extent to which these states have performed in changing the quality of human life measured by percapita income as well as some other indicators of human development based on available information.

Human development

Of late, United Nations' Development Programme [UNDP] has offered a broader perspective of human well-being which could offer an alternative to the prevailing notion of development. While recognizing income as an important objective, UNDP has emphasized improvements in non-income components of well-being, such as basic education and health. Education, good health, and other human attainments are valuable constituent determinants of our basic capabilities. These capabilities ultimately generate economic success as well as enhance the quality of human life [Sen: 1999].

Economic Growth and Human Development

Human development is now considered something additional to material advancement. There are instances of improvement in the sphere of human life without substantial improvement in material terms. The report published by the United Nations' Development Programme[1990] revealed that countries like Sri Lanka, Chile, Jamaika, Thailand, Tanzania, for example, did much better on their human development ranking. On the other hand, Oman, Saudi Arabia, Algeria, Senegal, have a much higher income ranking with considerably worse records on their human development. A study on Asian poverty reflects that China has done much better performance in terms of quality of life with similar level of gross national product [GDP] percapita to that of India and Pakistan [Bhattacharjee: 1998]. As such, it is not necessary that a population should be economically advanced as in western countries or urbanized largely, or employed mostly in non-agricultural sector in order to enjoy a better quality of life [Srinivasan : 1997]. The recent success in achieving certain goals of development in the states of Goa, Kerala and Tamil Nadu, also substantiate that a policy environment, which includes political will and strategic planning; bureaucratic efficiency, including management skills etc. can contribute a lot in changing the condition of society without substantial advancement in material front [Srinivasan : 1995]. Therefore, well-being of the people could be improved, and social, political and cultural conditions transformed, even at a low level of income, when there is appropriate public action [Ramchandran : 1999].

Gross Domestic Product and Per Capita Product

Although the limitations of income effect in achieving certain aspect of human development has been well documented, growth of domestic product (per capita) is widely used as a handy apparatus to indicate success in material advancement. Table 8.1 displays information regarding the growth of net domestic product as well as per capita GDP in the three states. A look at Table 8.1 reveals that the position of Tripura in this respect is the best. The increase in per capita income for Tripura during the last decade was nearly double than that of Assam. The increase in the growth of income was made possible in a condition when economic infrastructure and industrial base are no better in Tripura than in Assam. In terms of GDP and per capita income growth, Assam is in a dismal condition. The state could achieve merely 125.5 per cent against 238.83 per cent in Tripura and 165.20 per cent in Meghalaya.

Table 8.1
Three N.E.States : GDP and Per Capita Income

States	Gross Domestic Product			Per Capita Income		
	1990-91	2000-01	Growth %	1990-91	2000-01	Growth %
Assam	9775	26891	175.09	4432	10198	125.50%
Meghalaya	884	3230	265.38	4944	13114	165.20%
Tripura	1193	4580	283.90	4240	14348	238.83%

Source: Indian Economic Survey Report - 2002 - 2003.

Literacy

Rate of literacy is being used as an index of educational achievement. Literacy of three N.E.States are displayed in Table 8.2.

Table 8.2
Literacy Rate & Gender-gap in Literacy [2001] in Three NE States

States	Area	Male	Female	Gender Gap
Assam	Total	71.3	54.6	16.7
	Rural	68.2	50.7	17.6
	Urban	89.7	802	0.95
Meghalaya	Total	65.4	59.6	05.6
	Rural	59.2	53.2	06.6
	Urban	89.0	83.5	05.6
Tripura	Total	81.0	64.9	16.1
	Rural	78.4	60.5	17.9
	Urban	93.2	85.0	08.2

Source : Census Report of India - 2001.

The data presented in Table 8.2 indicate that urban male population in the three states has attained more than 85 per cent literacy. According to UNESCO, a state in which more than 85 per cent of the adult population is literate is called totally literate. However, urban female literacy is marginally lower. On the other hand, the rural scenario is not up to that extent where, the condition of female literacy is seriously lagging. This has raised the problem of gender-gap in literacy. The gender-gap in Assam and in Tripura is acute. The striking feature regarding the gender-gap in Meghalaya is that it has the least gender-gap. Gender-gap is a serious obstacle to development. Achievement of development goals becomes almost difficult where female education is neglected

Educational Infrastructure

Improvement of human resources and human skill are essential ingredients of human development. A society, which is unable to develop the skill and knowledge of its people, and to utilize them effectively, will be unable to develop. The principal mechanism for developing human skills and knowledge is the formal education system in a society [Toddaro : 1983]. The progress of education largely depends on existing educational infrastructure. Table 8.3 presents relative scenario of educational infrastructure.

Table 8.3
Number of Schools Per 1000 population in 2001 in Three NE States

States	Primary	Middle	High & H. S.
Assam	1.24	0.30	0.17
Meghalaya	2.03	0.45	0.29
Tripura	0.65	1.30	0.20
India	0.21	0.20	0.12

Source : Computed from Indian Economic Survey Report - 2002-2003.

Educational infrastructure as displayed in Table 8.3 reveals that the position of Meghalaya in respect of number of primary schools per thousand people is the best. Regarding the number of middle school, Tripura ranks first. Again in respect of High and higher secondary schools, the position of Meghalaya is the best. Position of educational infrastructure as indicated by the number of schools per thousand population presented in table 8.3 reveals that the three states are in a better position than the all Indian average. However, mere number of schools does not tell the entire story of infrastructure in education. Other aspects such as, student teacher ratio and amenities of education have significant bearing.

Enrolment Ratio

Enrolment ratio is another indicator regarding performance of the state in the field of education. A sharp fall in the enrolment ratio indicates increasing number of dropouts, which, in many cases, adds to the volume of child labour. Table 8.4 presents enrolment ratio in the three states only up to middle school.

Table 8.4
Gross Enrolment Ratio in Class I - V and VI-VIII [2001] in Three NE States

States	Enrolment			
	Class I-V		Class VI-VIII	
	Boys	Girls	Boys	Girls
Assam	125.44	106.44	80.02	63.67
Meghalays	118.79	110.41	59.04	62.35
Tripura	116.20	97.61	69.03	59.52

Source : Indian Economic Survey Report - 2002-2003

The data as displayed in Table 8.4 indicate that Assam tops in enrolment of boys into primary classes. Enrolment in primary classes in Tripura is the lowest. The position of Meghalaya in this field is somewhat different. Ratio of girls enrolled in primary classes is the highest. In case of enrolment in middle school, Assam tops the list. For Meghalaya a heavy dropout is marked regarding enrolment of boys. Gender-gap also persists in case of Tripura. Differential rates of enrolment of boys and girls at various levels are significant indicator of growing divide between them in terms of educational attainment.

Electrification and Safe Drinking Water

The essential indicators of good governance is its ability to provide basic amenities to households. Planners and policy makers have been striving hard to reallocate resources and device plans to provide quality life for the common people. The extent to which life of common man is becoming better in terms of availability of basic amentities like drinking water and provision of power supply is presented in Table 8.5

Table 8.5
Electrification and Safe drinking Water (2001) in Three NE States

States	Area	%of Households having access to electricit	Households having access to safe drinking Water			
			Sources	No. of Families	%of Families	Total
Assam	Total	24.90	Tap	459292	09.30	58.85%
	Rural	16.53	Hand pump	2201471	44.60	
	Urban	74.28	Tube Well	244379	04.95	
Meghalaya	Total	42.73	Tap	145096	34.52	39.94%
	Rural	30.26	Hand pump	8217	01.95	
	Urban	88.14	Tube well	10411	02.47	
Tripura	Total	41.84	Tap	162801	24.59	52.53%
	Rural	31.75	Hand pump	98403	14.86	
	Urban	86.36	Tube well	86612	13.08	

Source : Census Report of India 2001

Data as displayed in Table 8.5 reveal that the Meghalaya has the highest percentage of total households having access to electricity, following Tripura and Assam. On the other hand, Tripura has the highest percentage of rural households having access to electricity unlike other states. Regarding the source of drinking water, present study has taken tap, hand-pump, and tube-well as safe sources of drinking water. The data on source of water indicate that Assam has the highest percentage of households having access to safe drinking water. There is another dimension of the problem regarding the distance of the source of water. It may be within the premise, near the premise or away from the premise. For simplification, the distance of the households from the source of water is neglected. Nevertheless, distance of source of drinking water has significant bearing on human well-being. Another simplification is made in the form performance of the government of Assam, where it could ensure safe drinking water to a very meager percentage of households .

Material Aspect of Well-being

The conventional view of measuring material improvement is per capita income. However, the percapita income does not tell the entire story of well-being. Households' possession of specified assets might be taken as a proxy for material improvement. Table 8.6 presents the relevant information.

Table 8.6
Percentage of Households' access to specified service and possession of assets [2001] in Three NE States

States	Area	Banking Service	Radio/ Tran-sistor	Television	Telephone	Scooter/ Motor cycle	Car or van
Assam	Total	20.53	30.18	18.29	04.34	05.20	00.20
	Rural	14.97	28.60	12.04	01.88	03.31	01.15
	Urbar	53.29	39.49	55.21	18.85	16.36	07.33
Meghalaya	Total	20.82	31.96	20.88	05.95	02.89	02.69
	Rural	12.70	28.94	10.54	01.57	01.52	01.28
	Urbar	50.36	42.96	58.54	21.99	07.86	07.79
Tripura	Total	26.46	28.51	23.70	05.24	03.92	01.08
	Rural	20.63	25.61	15.04	09.10	01.96	00.77
	Urbar	52.15	41.28	59.96	19.25	12.55	02.47

Source : Computation Based on Census Report of India - 2001.

The information as presented in table 8.6 about households' possession of specified assets reveals that more than 50 per cent of urban household in the three states are availing banking service. Regarding rural counterparts, position of Tripura is the best where more than 20 per cent of the rural households are availing the service unlike other two states where much fewer percentage of households are exposed to banking service. Regarding the possession of electronic media, position of Tripura in respect of back dated media like radio and transistor is worse than the two other states but in terms of the modern means of media i.e.,television, position of Tripura is the best. As regards to telephone, there is no significant difference in Tripura, much great proportion of rural population is having telephone connection compared to Assam and Meghalaya. Coming to the question of possession of automobiles, Assam and Meghalaya's position are better than Tripura. It may be noted that the inequality in income distribution in Tripura is less pronounced than the other two states.

Conclusion

Human resource development is a key factor in the process of economic development. The success of any development strategy depends largely on the extent to which human resource is developed in terms of skill, education, health etc. Review of comparative performance in achieving human well-being in terms of a few indicators of human development is but a patch work. As human development depends on numerous factors including income and non-income components. Comprehensive survey of performance should include all those determining factors of human well-being. Nevertheless, review of this nature is effective in providing important insight into the nature of the problem of different regions for framing appropriate public action. To quote Noble Laureate Professor Amartya Sen, There are great many things that we can learn from within the country, by using the diversity of our experiences, particularly in the use of public action.' The comparative performance study can help focus the areas, where public action needs immediate address. The present review of performance experience in the referred states of northeastern India is directed to highlight the performance of the respective government in promulgating human well-being. The review has explored that in most cases the state of Tripura has done relatively better in many field of human development than the other two states. To conclude with the words of P. Mahanchandran, to make government development programme a success, it is important that factors associated with poor performance be identified. This would help policy makers to either reformulate the process or to adopt appropriate strategies for an effective implementation of the programmes in areas of less development.

REFERENCES

Bhattacharjee, Basabi [1998] : 'Urbanization and Human Development in West Bengal : A District Level Study and Comparison with inter state variation'. *Economic and Political Weekly*. Vol. XXXIII Nos. 47 &48, Nov. 21-27/28-Dec.4,1998.

Mahanchandran P.(1997): 'Interregional Comparison of Demographic Condition', *in Kerela's Demographic Transition–Determinates and Consequesnces*, edited by K.C. Zacharia and S. Irudaya Rajan.

Ramachandran, V. K. [1999] : 'On Kerala's Development' : in Jean Dreze and Amartya Sen, ed, *Indian Development–Selected Regional Perspectives*.

Sen, Amartya, [1999] : Radical Needs and Moderate Reform' : Indian Development - Selected Regional Perspectives. Jean Dreze and Amartya Sen.

Srinivasan, K. [1995]; 'Lessons from Goa, Karala and Tamin Nadu - The three Successful fertility Transition states in India, in *Demography India*. Vol-24, No. 2, 1995.

Todaro, Micheal P, [1983]: *Economic Development in the Third World.*

Statistical Facts: *Economic Survey of India* - 2002-03

Census Report of India - 2001; Office of the Registrar General, India

Statistical Abstract of Tripura - 2002 : Director of Economics and Statistics, Govt. of Tripura.

Some Basic Statistics - 2002 : Director of Economics and Statistics, Govt. of Tripura.

Tripura at a Glance - 2001 : Director of Economics and Statistics, Govt. of Tripura.

9

DATA OF HIGHER EDUCATION FOR HUMAN RESOURCE DEVELOPMENT IN NORTH EAST INDIA

– *K.S. Chakraborty*

Higher Education conventionally refers to the studies beyond school level. Universities, Colleges and other institutions of higher learning are its main constituents. In our country, despite a marked increase in the number of such institution, performance of many are not up to expectations due to shortage of funds, high costs, imprudent utilization of resources, improper planning, unsustainable increase in enrolment for higher studies etc. (Chakraborty : 1997) The present scenario is further characterized by non-availability of data in a manner, which are comparable as well as compatible. North East India is no exception. In view of the continuing backwardness of the region the need for a new and synergetic incentive package to stimulate overall development is widely felt. Since the last decade the Governments, both Central and States, have been taking a keen interest in the industrial development of this region. We know natural resources of this region are abundant yet scarcity is felt in terms of efficient manpower. The success of higher education in providing efficient manpower is, however, contingent upon proper planning for which adequate data are required (Chakraborty and Haldar : 1998). If there are deficiencies in the machanism of providing data on regular basis, the potentiality of higher education to contribute to development would be seriously inspired (Mehata : 1993).

In this backdrop, the present chapter focuses upon the issues associated with data of higher education in the north eastern region of India. The quality of information and data is a pre-requisite for planning of educational activities. In brief, quality data provide adequate information to educational planners, administrators, authorities, researchers etc. for policy prescriptions and decision making.

Present Data Sources of Higher Education

The data on higher education of the North East Region may be collected either from the national level agencies or specific state / regional agencies. There are two main agencies which collect statistics in higher education namely, University Grants Commission and the Planning, Monitoring and Statistical Division of the Ministry of Human Resource Development (MHRD) on regular basis. Apart from these, the Association of Indian Universities (AIU) and National Institute of Educational Planning and Administration (NIEPA) are also important agencies for providing data on higher education. Of late, the National Assessment and Accreditation Council (NACC) publishes data on the accredited organizations of higher studies.

The office of the Registrar General of India provides information on population statistics as also on many items through its Census of India publications. The National Sample Survey Organisation (NSSO) and the Central Statistical Organisations (CSO) also collect and publish statistics on sample basis. The apex educational institution like ICSSR, collect data on education occasionally through their research projects and surveys.

Another important data collecting source in this region is

the North Eastern Council (NEC) which publishes Basic Statistics of each north eastern state and the region as a whole. The available data is limited to the enrolment figures, number of educational institutions as well as budget expenditure on higher education. The Statistical Department of all the north eastern states also come up with similar publications.

Problems with the Present Data System

Major difficulties which the educational planners, administrators and the users of these data face with regard to data on education are numerous. As stated, there exists multiple sources of educational statistics but there is no coordination between them which often gives different results for the same item creating severe comparability problems. e.g. there is a difference between the data published by NEC and that of the Statistics Department, Government of Tripura regarding the educational statistics. Secondly, the date of reference of the educational data may vary from source to source. e.g. it is found that while higher educational institutes make general education data available according to the academic calendar year, the budget and expenditure data is available according to the financial year. Thirdly, quite a significant problem is the time lag in educational data. Different volumes of publications are available for different years while provisional / selective data is made available for the time being. In the Basic Statistics 2000, the data on the number of educational institutions is shown as on September, 1996. Fourthly, due to administrative adjustment time and again boundaries of state / districts change making it difficult to construct a time series required for decentralized planning. e.g in Tripura, a new district has been created recently which limits the comparability of data in the district level. Fifthly, data users face certain problems unique to educational information, inadequate sampling techniques, checking procedures, defects in reporting agencies, coverage gaps etc. Sixthly, to top all such bottlenecks, the educational planner finds absolutely no data on unit cost, teaching cost, tution cost, number of unrecognized institutions, teachers by age and qualifications, enrolment by sex caste and family income distribution of establishments by capacity / size / space of class rooms, non-formal or correspondence courses, accessibility to media/computers, drop-out rates etc.Time series of these data are absolutely necessary for long term planning.

Uses of Higher Education Data

Efficiency of the organisation to a certain extent depends upon the regularity of information based on accurate data. As a matter of fact, the ultimate effectiveness of the information is itself dependent upon the users for whom data is required. In the context of higher education, it is, perheps not an exaggeration to assume that the government, UGC or any other agency which provide fund for higher educational establishments have every right to know how efficiently the fund is being used. Likewise students, parents or researchers may be other users of the data (NAAC : 1996). To the users, it is very much significant that the data should be pertinent and meaningful. Generation of such data involves identifying the purpose for which it will be used (Hawkings : 1972). The following are the significant purposes for which data may be required.

(i) to provide information to government, UGC or any other funding agency regarding the utilization of funds, wastage, performance etc.

(ii) to provide data to students regarding the academic or extra-academic achievements,

(iii) to give data to parents about cost and quality of education.

(iv) to supply information to researchers in the area of interest.

(v) to give information to the staff about significant events,

(vi) to provide information to educational policy maker for decision making.

(vii) to report on activities which has social impact in general.

Publication of Annual Report as Data Bank

The Educational Planners require data on population by sex, area, economic levels, density etc. The status of literacy, distribution of habitation related to districts / educational blocks/ towns are also required. Undoubtedly, the quality of information depends upon the needs and expectations of the users. Collection of quality data on higher education in North-east is possible only if all the establishments of higher studies provide data in prescribed form on regular basis. Publication of Annual Reports by the establishment of higher studies is one of the ideal source of information. A suggestive model of Annual Report may be constructed in the following manner.

All data relating to an establishment cannot be disclosed in annual reports because that would make reports too large, costly and sometimes confusing. Information which is meaningful and capable of effective judgement must be taken into consideration. Relevance, thus, should be treated as the primary qualitative objective of annual report (Saeed : 1990). In view of the above, the following are the relevant information to be disclosed in the annual report of establishments of higher studies:

1. Data on academic affairs.
2. Data on extra academic affairs.
3. Data on financial affairs.
4. Head of the Institution's Report.
5. An abstract of basic information.

Data on academic affairs may include number of students at different stages, number of teachers department wise, the teacher student ratio, percentage of successful candidates in the final exams with proportion of first and second class holders, success of honours students, academic distinctions like scholarships, awards and medals won at the university examinations, research activities, academic achievements of the teachers etc.

Data on extra-academic affairs may include participation as well as distinctions obtained in NC.C., N.S.S. activities, sports, drama, quizzes, debates etc.

Data on financial affairs may include :

(a) receipts and payments account for the year,

(b) income and expenditure account for the year,

(c) a balance sheet as on specified date,

(d) a statement of annual cost per student.

The Receipts and Payment Account shows money received and paid for various items during the year. While Income and Expenditure account includes only the amounts relevant for the year under reference adjusted for arrears and advances. Transactions on capital account are completely excluded from this account. The cost of education per student includes expenditure on guardian's share towards books, stationary and others. It may also include government expenditure on supervision, inspection and policy making.

Head of the Institution's Report : The report should discuss mainly the role of the educational institution in the society and special performance of that institution. The report should also include the reasons affecting the performance of the students in academic or extra-curricular activities, further plans of action for improving quality, introduction of new courses, extension of research facilities, introduction of computer, equipment for laboratory, explain the future development plans etc.

An Abstract of some basic information may include the following:

(a) Library books per student,

(b) Teacher cost per student

(c) Salary cost per student
(d) Fee cost per student
(e) Total expenditure per student
(f) Capital expenditure per student
(g) Expenditure on co-curricular activities per student
(h) Internal source of finance per students
(i) External sources of finance per student.

In order to facilitate the user, the above data need to be incorporated in the annual reports in appropriate form structured logically and the key points be highlighted. It will no doubt facilitate comparison so essential for educational planning methods. Such a comprehensive annual reporting system will integrate all the activities of the higher education of a district, a state and link it to all the North Eastern states. This Annual Reporting System may serve as a support system to the planning, organizing and monitoring functions of higher education department. This may be a system for retrieving data and information to analyse and make available for utilization.

Conclusion

The basic idea of annual reporting by educational institutions of the North-East emphasises on the generation of data. But the educational establishment can only act in this direction if there is legal provision, like corporate reporting practices in India is largely guided by the Indian Companies Act. In educational institutions a uniform law should be deviced for practice of keeping the users informed through the mechanism of submission of annual reports. Most of the institutions of higher studies in North-Eastern India get financial support and recognition from the U.G.C. (NERO) besides central and state governments. Therefore UGC (NERO) may frame appropriate rules for publishing the annual reports for each academic year before sanctioning any grant to the establishments. Moreover, NEC may also issue directive and provide fund to the establishments of higher studies in North East India.

REFERENCES

Chakraborty, K.S : "TQM Concept in Higher Education of India", Vidyasagar University Journal of commerce, Vol.2, March, 1997, pp. 31-35.

Chakraborty, K.S and Halder P.K.: "Re-engineering Higher Education in India," Business Studies, Department of Commerce, Calcutta University, Vol. XXI, July,1998, pp. 54-57.

Hawkings, David F. : *Financial Reporting Practices of Corporations*, Dow Jones - Irwin, Homewood, Illinois, 1972.

Mehata, B.C.: "Financing of Higher Education" *Journal of Educational Planning and Administratration*, Vol.VII, No.1, Jan -1993, New Delhi-, pp. 63-74.

National Assessment and Accreditation Council : *Quality Education through self-study and External Evaluation*, Bangalore, pp. 1-3.

Saved, M. (Edited) : *Corporate Financial Reporting*, Anmol Publications, New Delhi, 1990.

10

HUMAN RESOURCE DEVELOPMENT IN MANIPUR : A DISCLAIMER

– K. Gyanendra Singh

Human development is a process of enlarging people's choices. It is not just choices among different detergents, television channels, or car models but the choices that are created by expanding human capabilities and functionings - what people do and can do in their lives. But at all levels of development, the three essential ones are: to lead a long and healthy life, to acquire knowledge and to have access to resources needed for a decent standard of living (HDR : 1990).

Human development deals with creating conditions that enable people to get the best out of themselves and their lives. Development is a never-ending process. Human development has two sides - the formation of human capabilities such as improved health, knowledge and skills and the use people make of their acquired capabilities for leisure, productive purposes or being active in cultural, social and political affairs.

There are three key indicators of human resource development. The first component is longevity - life expectancy at birth. The use of life expectancy as one of the indicators rests on three considerations - the intrinsic value of longevity, its value in helping people pursue various goals and its association with other characteristics, such as good health and nutrition.

The second key component is knowledge - literacy figures are only a crude reflection of access to education, particularly to the good quality education so necessary for productive life in modern society.

The third key component is command over resources, needed for a decent living.

But these three key indicators suffer from a common failing - they are averages that conceal wide disparities in the overall population. Different social groups have different life expectancies. There often are wide disparities in male and female literacy and income is distributed unevenly.

Educational Attainments

Education is perhaps the single most important means to improve personal endowments, build capability levels, overcome constraints and in the process enlarge available set of opportunities and choices for a sustained improvement in well-being. It is a life-long process. It starts from the cradle and ends at the grave for an individual. Education is important not merely as a means to other ends, but it is an attribute that is valued in itself, by most individuals. More importantly, it is a critical invasive instrument for bringing about social, economic and political inclusion and a durable integration of people, particularly those 'excluded' from the mainstream of any society. Creation, application and adaptation of new technologies; lower fertility, infant and child mortality rate; better nutritional, hygience and health status of children, reproductive health and empowerment of women; social mobility and political freedom, all have visible linkages with educational attainments of people (HDR : 1999). It is, undoubtedly, a basic component of human development. Some Educational Indicators of Manipur are discused below.

i) Literacy Rate

The Census of India currently defines the literacy rate as proportion of literates to total population in the age group 7 years and above.

The literacy rate increased from 49.66 per cent in 1981 to 59.85 per cent in 2001 in Manipur. The all India rate is 43.5 per cent in 1981 and it increased to 55.18 per cent in 2001. Manipur is performing more or less at par with the national average (Table 10.1).

Table 10.1
Literacy Rate in Manipur (percentage)

Year		Manipur	India
1981	M	64.15	56.38
	F	34.67	29.76
	P	49.66	43.57
1991	M	71.63	64.13
	F	47.60	39.29
	P	59.89	52.21
2001	M	67.58	63.98
	F	51.95	45.75
	P	59.85	55.18

Source : National HDR 2001, Planning Commission, Govt. of India, March 2002, Oxford, and basic Statistics of NER 2002, Govt. of India, NEC Secretariat, Shillong.

ii) Adult Literacy Rate

The adult literacy rate, in India, is defined as the proportion of literate population in age group 15 years and above. It gives an indication of stock of human capital in population.

In Manipur, the proportion of adult literates in the population increased from 47.04 per cent in 1981 to 64.49 per cent in 1995-96. In India, it increased from 40.83 per cent in 1981 to 54.32 per cent in 1995-96 (Table 10.2).

Table 10.2
Adult Literacy Rate in Manipur : 1995-96 (percentage)

	Manipur	India
M	76.03	67.25
F	52.29	40.67
P	64.49	54.32

Source : National HDR 2001, Planning Commission, Govt. of India, March 2002, Oxford.

iii) Age-Specific Enrolment Ratio

It refers to percentage of children enrolled in a particular age group, irrespective of the level/class of enrolment, to the total population of children in that age group. However, it suffers from a limitation that it does not give the schooling level/class at which the students are enrolled.

For age group 6-11 years, there is a decline from 50.7 per cent in 1981 to 48.2 per cent in 1991 in case of Manipur but it registered an increase from 47.2 per cent in 1981 to 51.2 per cent in 1991 in case of national average. For age group 11-14 years, it registered an increase of 64.4 per cent in 1981 to 71.9 per cent in 1991. In India also it increased from 50.5 per cent in 1981 to 62.1 per cent in 1991 (Table 10.3).

Table 10.3
Age-Specific Enrolment Ratios in Manipur (percentage)

		Manipur	India
Age group 6 to below 11 years	1981	50.7	47.2
	1991	48.1	51.2
Age group 11 to below 14 years	1981	67.4	50.0
	1991	71.9	62.1

Source : National HDR 2001, Planning Commission, Govt. of India, March 2002, Oxford.

iv) Intensity of Formal Education - Adjusted

This indicator is based on class-wise enrolment rates and it attempts to capture current progress in spread of formal education among school going children. It implicitly takes care of the drop out rates across all classes. The adjusted intensity of formal education has a higher value for states that are able to have higher level of enrolment in higher classes or in other words are able to retain children in schools for a longer duration without dropping out and at the same time have a larger proportion of children of school going age-group, enrolled in schools.

At national level, the adjusted intensity of formal education was estimated at 2.04 years in 1978 and it increased to 2.70 years in 1993. In Manipur, it was estimated at 2.80 years in 1978 and 3.64 years in 1993 (Table 10.4).

Table 10.4
Intensity of Formal Education in Manipur - Adjusted

	1978			1993		
	R	U	T	R	U	T
Manipur	2.34	4.97	2.80	3.07	5.16	3.64
India	1.68	3.20	2.04	2.31	3.81	2.70

Source : National HDR 2001, Planning Commission, Govt. of India, March 2002, Oxford

These indicators show that Manipur has performed very well in case of educational attainments.

Health Attainments

Not much is known regarding health attainments in Manipur due to non-availability of data. But some inference can be drawn from the infant mortality rate.

IMR is defined as number of death by age 1 per 1000 live births. In Manipur it has declined from 32 per thousand in 1981 to 28 per thousand in 1991. The all India rate also declined from 115 per thousand in 1981 to 77 per thousand in 1991. (Table 10.5)

Table 10.5
Infant Mortality Rate in Manipur (per thousand)

	1981			1991		
	M	F	P	M	F	P
Manipur	31	33	32	29	27	28
India	122	108	115	74	79	77

Source : National HDR 2001, Planning Commission, Govt. of India, March 2002, Oxford.

Economic Attainments and Well-Being

To capture an individual's command over resources, as well as the opportunities and attainments in other aspects of well-being, per capita consumption expenditure is used. This has been adjusted for inequality using Gini Ratios estimated from the respective consumption expenditure.

In Manipur, the inequality adjusted per capita consumption expenditure was at Rs. 101.16 per month in 1983 and it increased to Rs. 476.02 per month in 1999-2000. The all India average was Rs. 86.59 per month in 1983 and it increased to Rs. 418.18 in 1999-2000 (Table 10.6).

Table 10.6
Inequality Adjusted Per Capita Consumption Expenditure in Manipur (fig. in Rupees per month)

	1983	1993-94	1999-2000
Manipur	101.06	259.64	476.02
India	86.59	228.69	418.18

Source : National HDR 2001, Planning Commission, Govt. of India, March 2002, Oxford

Employment Indicators

The level of employment, its composition and the growth in employment opportunities are critical indicators of the process of economic development in any economy. These are also indicators that directly capture the economic attainments and hence the level of well being of the people.

It is estimated as compound annual growth in the persons employed in the age group 15 years and above on the usual principal and subsidiary status. The growth of employment declined from 3.3 per cent in 1983 to 1993-94 to 2 per cent in 1993-94 to 1999-2000. The all India rate also declined from 2.1 per cent in 1983 to 1993-94 to 1.6 per cent in 1993-94 to 1999-2000 (Table 10.7).

Table 10.7

Growth In Employment in Manipur (percent per annum)

	1983 to 1993-94			1993-94 to 1999-2000		
	M	F	P	M	F	P
Manipur	3.6	2.9	3.3	3.2	-0.3	2.0
India	2.2	1.7	2.1	1.9	0.9	1.6

Source : National HDR 2001, Planning Commission, Govt. of India, March 2002, Oxford.

The incidence of unemployment is defined as the percentage of persons unemployed in the age group 15 years and above on the usual principal and subsidiary status to the total number of persons in the labour force. The incidence of unemployment increased from 0.4 per cent in 1983 to 3.5 per cent in 1999-2000. The all India rate also increased from 2 per cent in 1983 to 2.3 per cent in 1999-2000 (Table 10.8).

Table 10.8

Incidence of Unemployment in Manipur (as a percentage of labour force)

	1983	1993-94	1999-2000
Manipur	0.4	1.8	3.5
India	2.0	2.0	2.3

Source : National HDR 2001, Planning Commission, Govt. of India, March 2002, Oxford.

The HDI shows that the rank of Manipur has declined from 4th rank in 1981 to 9th rank in 1991. The HDI is a composite of variables capturing attainments in three dimensions of human development viz., economic, educational and health. These have been captured by per capita monthly expenditure adjusted for inequality; a combination of literacy rate and intensity of formal education and a combination of life expectancy at age 1 and infant mortality rate (Table-10.9).

Table 10.9
Human Development Index of Manipur

		Rural		Urban		Combined	
		Value	Rank	Value	Rank	Value	Rank
	1981	0.44	2	0.553	5	0.461	4
Manipur	1991	0.503	7	0.618	12	0.536	9
	1981	0.263		0.442		0.302	
India	1991	0.340		0.511		0.381	

Source : National HDR 2001, Planning Commission, Govt. of India, March 2002, Oxford.

These observations give a very contrasting picture. Manipur is highly ranked in HDI. It has performed well in case of educational attainments, health (though much information is not available) and economic attainments to some extent. But when it comes to employment indicators, it gives a very grim picture. As already pointed out, human development has two sides - formation of human capabilities and the use of these capabilities for productive purposes. If we look at the above indicators we can say that manipur has done well only in one side, i.e., formation of human capabilities such as improved health and knowledge. But it has failed in the other side, i.e., it has failed to use these acquired health and knowledge for productive purposes. One example is the rising unemployment among the educated youth.

Table 10.10

Registration and Placing Done Through Employment Exchanges in Manipur

Year	No. of registrants on the live register	Growth rate (%)	No. of persons placed in appointments
1980-81	115546	—	703
1982-83	153691	33.01	955
1983-84	176931	15.12	664
1984-85	194581	9.07	638
1985-86	237179	21.89	402
1986-87	266694	12.44	537
1987-88	249074	–6.61	1909
1988-89	248438	–0.26	226
1989-90	254310	2.36	292
1990-91	183495	–27.85	242
1991-92	198148	7.99	174
1992-93	215677	8.85	310
1993-94	241272	11.87	1390
1994-95	249910	3.58	1085
1995-96	276157	10.50	143
1996-97	299881	8.59	579
1997-98	322253	7.46	429
1998-99	354269	9.94	162
1999-2000	387890	9.49	69
2000-01	397304	2.43	2
2001-02	409652	3.11	—
2002-03	417338	1.88	5

Source : Statistical Handbooks of Manipur, 1992 and 2002.

From Table 10.10 we see that the number of registrants in the live register is increasing every year. Whereas the placement done is decreasing and in the past two-three years the number of persons placed in appointments is almost nil compared to the number of registrants in the live register.

If we look at the distribution of working population (Table 10.11), we see that about 70 per cent of its population is engaged in primary sector, about 10 per cent in secondary sector and about 20 per cent in tertiary sector. Working population in secondary sector has actually declined from about 13 per cent in 1981 to about 10 per cent in 1991. This shows that the public sector has become stagnant and there are no job opportunities in the public sector. Educated youth are unlikely to seek jobs in the primary sector. Again, working in tertiary sector requires certain skills. So, we have to create a type of self-employment situation in order to absorb the educated unemployed (Das and Singh : 2004). But such a situation is not seen in Manipur. Then the question arises where the fault lies ?

Table 10.11
Distribution of Working Population by Industry in Manipur

Industry	**1971**	**1981**	**1991**
Primary Sector	264421	399033	495792
	(71.30%)	(69.60%)	(70%)
Secondary Sector	45361	76568	68404
	(12.23%)	(13.35%)	(9.66%)
Tertiary Sector	61081	97738	144087
	(16.47%)	(17.05%)	(20.34%)
Total Main Workers	370863	573339	708283
Total Population	1072753	1420953	1837149

Source: Census of India, 1971, Manipur, General Economic Tables, Series-12, Part II-B, Census of India, 1981, India, general Economic tables, Series-I, Part II-A and Statistical Handbook of Manipur, 1992.

We can argue that this is because our educational system is still in its traditional form. It is lacking behind in imparting good quality education and it has failed to impart that type of education where there is skill-formation.

Every year the number of educational institutions is increasing. With the rise in population, the enrolment rate in these institutions is also increasing. But the question is where do these people go after they passed from these institutions ?

It is not enough for countries simply to grant economic and social rights in theory only. We cannot legislate good health and jobs. We need an economy strong enough to provide them and for that we need people economically engaged. People will work because they enjoy the fruits of their labour - fair pay, education and health care for their families and so forth. They will build the wealth that allows them to be compensated. But if the rewards are denied, they will lose their motivation. And this is what is happening in Manipur. Poeple have lost their motivation, especially the educated youth. The denial of job opportunities to these people, i.e., educated youth has led to youth unrest in Manipur. We can say that this may be one of the factors which have led to the mushrooming of insurgent activities in the state (Das and Singh : 2004). This has also led to alcoholism and drug addiction. It is really surprising that Manipur, which has done very well in case of educational attainments, has the maximum number of drug addicts and HIV positive cases.

REFERENCES

Basic Statistics of NER 2002, Govt. of India, NEC Secretariat, Shillong Das, Gurudas and K. Gyanendra Singh, 2004, *Unemployment in Manipur : Some Policy Implications,* presented in the seminar on "Educated youth and Unemployment in Manipur" organized by EGERC, Manipur and sponsored by ICSSR, New Delhi on 24-25 June, 2004.

Human Development Report 1990, UNDP

Ibid., 1999, UNDP

National Human Development Report 2001, Planning Commission, Govt. of India, March 2002.

11

DIMENSION OF HUMAN RESOURCE DEVELOPMENT IN NORTH EAST INDIA: THE CASE OF MIZORAM

– *R. Lalnun Tluanga*

Human Capital

Economic growth and development is the result of many factors. However, the contribution of human capital has gained ground only in recent years. It has now been central point of development planning of any country. By human capital, we mean the 'sum total of the knowledge, skills and aptitudes of the people, inhabiting the country. Broadly, it includes the initiative, resourcefulness, capacity for sustained work, right values, interest and attitudes and all other human qualities conducive to higher output and accelerated economic growth'. This implies that a country having the largest population is not necessarily the richest in human capital. Many of the very densely populated countries of Asian region are the most deficient in human capital. The most important resource in the world consists of education, experience, skill, health, etc. of the people. Schultz thinks of population quality as derived from two sources, namely, genetic endowment and acquired abilities. Of the two, acquired abilities seem to play a more important role for economic growth and development of a country. The genes inherent in different population, of course, are not the same, it is not responsible much for the difference in abilities and efficiency in different countries.

For an accelerated economic growth and development it is necessary to improve the quality of the population. Increased investment in physical capital alone will not bring much change unless there is improvement in human skills and knowledge. In fact, advances in knowledge and skills made a vast improvement in physical capital which, in turn, affect economic growth. It is now widely believed that development of human quality through education, training and health care etc. has a very important role to play in achieving self-sustaining economic development. The developing countries have, therefore, become increasingly conscious of the need for developing human resources as part of national economic development.

Economic growth and development in modem time is generally brought about by scientific and technological advancement, that brings about a systematic improvement in equipment, machines and tools. For proper utillsation of these machines and other equipment, it is necessary to improve the skill and knowledge possessed by man. However, scientific and technological improvement cannot be evolved without proper training and education of the labour force. A country may be rich in natural and physical capital resources, but unless there are men who can mobilise, organise and harness nature's bountiful resources for the production of goods and services, no country can make progress towards economic and social advancement. Thus, the fundamental problem of the developing countries is, therefore, not so much the creation of wealth but rather the creation of the capacity to create wealth (Mehta : 1976).

The North East India

The development of human resources is a central objective of all development efforts. The proper utilisation of human resources provides the key to economic and social development. With this perspective in mind, the present study reviews the major trends and the present situation in the sphere of development and utilisation of human resources in the North-East with special emphasis on Mizoram, a small north eastern state of India. An attempt is also made here to present the progress made in respect of some of the important indicators of quality of life.

To appraise the economic condition of the North-East states, it is important to understand the distinctive characteristics of the region. The North Eastern Region consists of 7 states, viz, Arunachal Pradesh, Assam, Manipur, Meghalaya, Mizoram, Nagaland and Tripura. The region is small but strategically important because it is bounded by China and Bhutan, in the north, Burma in the east and Bangladesh in the south west, having a long stretch of international boundary. The total area of the region is 255039 sq. km which is 7.77 per cent of the whole country. With the exception of Assam and Arunachal Pradesh, all the states are small in size. Tripura is the smallest in size with 10,486 sq. km. Nagaland became a full-fledged state in 1963. Meghalaya was formed with two hill districts of Garo Hills and United Khasi and Jaintia Hills of Assam in 1970. Under the North Eastern Reorganisation Act, 1971, Meghalaya, Manipur and Tripura were given statehood, Arunachal and Mizorarn were also made Union Territories and further elevated to the status of state in February, 1987.

The topography of the North Eastern Region is characterised by undulating hilly terrain. Land under cultivation in the region is only 16 per cent of its total geographical area. It varies from 2.5 per cent in Arunachal Pradesh to 7.2 per cent in Manipur, 9.4 per cent in Meghalaya, 4 per cent in Mizoram, 15 per cent in Nagaland, 36 per cent in Tripura and 45 per cent in Assam (Bhattacharjee and Upadhaya : 2002). Population is scattered mainly in hill tops. This makes connectivity in terms of roads, communication, water supply and electricity very expensive. Needless to say, construction of roads becomes extremely arduous and costs almost twice compared to the plains. Due to its geographical isolation and the poor condition of roads any item brought from elsewhere in the country to the region naturally costs more. Likewise, any kind of produce put to sale outside the states also costs more. The total population of the region is about 3849 million, representing 3.74 per cent of total population of the country. The distribution of population is uneven, while Assam accommodates a little over 69 per cent of the population of the region, Mizoram shares only about 2.31 per cent. The region's decadal growth rate of population 22.02 is higher than the national average of 21.34. It is interesting to note that the two most populous states of the region Assam and Tripura record the lowest decennial growth rate at 18.85 and 15.74 respectively. The growth rate of Nagaland is surprisingly high at 64.41. The percentage of urban population to total population varies from 12.72 in Assam to 49.50 in Mizoram. It is noteworthy that except Mizoram, all other states of the region are below the national percentage of urbanisation at 27.78 according to 2001 census.

One striking aspect of the North Eastern Region is the constitutional safeguard especially provided to hill areas relating to land and tax. Income tax which is a burdensome responsibility does not pose problems for the tribals residing in the hill states of Arunachal, Meghalaya, Mizoram and Nagaland and hill areas of Assam, Manipur and Tripura as these people are exempted from income tax. The special provision is also made so that land cannot be sold to non-tribals. Manufacturing sector is relatively weak and insignificant in the region. Tertiary sector which is dominated by public administration and other services contribute most to the Net State Domestic Product. Except in Assam and in the plains of Manipur and Tripura, income from these sources do not come under the purview of tax net. Moreover, income from agriculture is also not captured. Consequently, these factors limit the tax base to a considerable extent in the region.

A Brief Survey of Mizoram

Mizoram is a hill state located in the north east corner of India, sandwiched between Myanmar and Bangladesh. Its total area is 21,081 sq. km with a total population of 8,91,058 (2001 census) which constitutes only 0.64 per cent of India's total area and 0.09 per cent of the total population of India. Out of the total population, 4,59,783 are male and 4,31,275 are female. The urban population constitutes 49.49 per cent. The decadal growth rate declined from 48.55 in 1971-1981 to 39.70 in 1981-1991 and further to 29 in 1991-2001. The density of population increased to 42 in 2001 from 33 in 1991. The whole state is composed of several ranges of hills which one separated from one another by narrow deep river valleys. There are a few and small patches of flat land between hill ranges.

Mizoram has an abundant growth of vegetation. About 85 per cent of the total area is under forest cover of either dense forest or open forest. Important forest produce mostly in the form of raw materials are bamboo, timber, 'firewood and charcoal, sungrass, broomsticks, cane, sand, stone and poles.

Mizoram is an agricultural state where majority of the population is engaged in agricultural activities. According to 2001 census, the proportion of workers to the population stood at 52.70 per cent. Out of the total workers, 54.83 per cent live in rural areas with a female share of 43.74 per cent. Cultivators dominate the working group contributing 53.91 per cent. The work participation rate has increased from 48.9 per cent in 1991 to 52.7 per cent in 2001, Shifting cultivation continues to be the principal and prevalent method of cultivation.

Education

Education is a key factor and an engine of development and social modernisation. The Constitution of India, in its directive principle also lays down that it is obligatory for the state government to provide universal and free primary education to the citizen. Realising the important role of education for all round development, the Third Five Year Plan emphasised the role of education thus "education is the single most important factor in achieving rapid economic development and technological progress and in creating social order founded on the values of freedom, social justice and equal opportunity. Programmes of education lie at the base of the effort to forge the bonds of common citizenship, to harness the energies of the people, and to develop the natural and human resources of every part of the country.

The National Policy on Education (NPE), 1986, and its Programme of Action (POA), as reviewed in 1992, envisaged improvement and expansion of education in all sectors, a stress on improvement in quality and relevance of education at all levels, along with technical and professional education. The goal of education policy is to provide education for all, giving prior importance to free and compulsory primary education to children in the age group of 6-14 years (upto standard V), total eradication of illiteracy, vocationalisation of education, covering children with special needs, special focus on education of women, weaker section and minorities.

In line with this policy, a high priority has been accorded to education in Mizoram by increasing expenditure on this sector every successive plan practically right from the state joined planning process after it became Union Territory in 1972. Total government expenditure on revenue account has shown a regular and secular trend, increasing in absolute as well as in percentage terms. During the Fifth Plan, a total of Rupees 22.74 crores was spent on education which was 12.96 per cent of total revenue expenditure. This increased to Rs. 56.96 crores with 13.16 per cent in the Sixth Plan. In the succeeding Seventh, Eight and Ninth plans, an increasing percentage of expenditure on revenue account has been incurred at the rate of 13.86 per cent, 16.32 per cent and 17.78 per cent to total revenue expenditure respectively. Out of this expenditure, elementary education has received the highest priority over the years.

The number of schools imparting primary and middle level of education in the state was 2050 in 2000-2001. The total number of pupils enrolled in these institutions were 1,50,842 during 2000-2001 as against 1,57,136 in the previous year. The institutions imparting high school and higher secondary level of education were 407 with a total number of students enrolled 46,686 during 2000-01 as against 388 with a total number of students enrolled 44,091 during 1999-2000. Out of these 2457 schools, 1562 are run by the state government, 307 are deficit schools and 135 are government aided schools. The remaining 453 are privately managed. Besides, there are quite a number of private english medium schools mainly managed by Churches and individuals as private institutions at primary and middle level of education. During 2000-01, there were 378 number of such schools with a total enrolment of 28,011. Adult education programme is also taken up seriously. Upto 2000- 01, the state government ran 40 number of Nodal Continuing Education Centres, 360 number of Continuing Education Centres and 400 number of libraries. Besides, SCERT provides academic and technical support for a qualitative improvement of school education.

Higher & Technical Education

There has been impressive growth in the number of institution and enrolment in higher education. There are at present 33 colleges and other higher educational institutions in the state. Out of these, 26–colleges are imparting general education like Arts, Science and Commerce. There are 2 number of Polytechnic, one law college and one college of Teachers' Education. The remaining 2 institutions are Hindi Training College. In addition to these, the state is now having a Central University.

In respect of higher technical education, the scope for pursuing higher education within the state is very limited. A college of Veterinary Science and Animal Husbandry imparting undergraduate courses of 5 years duration was recently established in Aizawl. Other institutions established in the state are ITI and Paramedical and Nursing college offering B.Sc. Nursing degree

Pharmacy course at diploma level and Certificate Course on Medical Lab Technology. As there is no college for studying medicine, forestry, agriculture, engineering etc., in Mizoram, students are sent to pursue various disciplines of higher technical education in the institutions of other states of the country. A number of students are sponsored by the state government through seat quota allotted to the state by different institutions. In addition to these, Indira Gandhi National Open University Regional Centre was established at Aizawl.

Literacy

The progress of literacy rates in Mizoram since 1951 is shown in Table 11.1. It exhibits that the literacy rate for the state as a whole increased from 31.14 per cent in 1951 to 88.49 per cent in 2001 with literacy rate for males at 90.69 per cent and that for females at 86.13 per cent. The highest increase of literacy rate in any one decade was recorded from 1981 to 1991 with an over all increase of 22.39 percentage points. The rate of increase during the same decade for male was 21.15 percentage points

Table- 11.1

Literacy Rate in Mizoram (in Percentage)

Year	Persons	Male	Female
1	2	3	4
1951	31.14	46.15	16.70
1961	44.01	53.40	34.69
1971	53.80	60.48	46.70
1981	59.88	64.45	54.91
1991	82.26	85.60	78.60
2001	88.49	90.69	86.13

Source : Census of India, various issues

Note : Literacy percentage for 1951,1961 and 1971 relate to population aged five years and above.

The Rates for the 1981 to 2001 relate to population aged seven years and above.

whereas female recorded 23.70. It is interesting to note that the growth rate of literacy has been higher in case of females than their male counterparts all through the years since 1951 to 2001. It is also encouraging to note that the growth rate of literacy in case of females from 16.70 per cent in 1951 to 86.13 per cent in 2001 was one of the highest in the country. The gap in male-female literacy rates has decreased from 29.45 percentage points in 1951 to 4.56 percentage points in 2001.

The aims of National Literacy Mission to achieve full literacy level of 75 per cent by the end of the year 2005 has been already achieved in Mizoram. Under the scheme of Sarva Shiksha Abhiyan, a massive campaign has been underway to achieve full literacy within the next two to three years.

Health and Family Welfare

Good and sound health is a pre-requisite for happy living. For an improved quality of life, primary health care has been accepted as one of the main instruments of action In the overall health care programme, emphasis has been laid on preventive and promotional' aspects and organising effective and efficient health services which are comprehensive in nature and easily and widely available, freely accessible and generally affordable by the people While a sound health is important for efficient working and happy life, on the contrary, ill- health is a hindrance and a retarding factor to progress.

Poverty and malnutrition are sinister twins responsible for depressed physical activity and low productivity in a backward economy. It is therefore vitally important to promote policies for stepping up medical and health services and human resource development. A healthy body and a sound mind constitute the most enduring and valuable economic assets that releases the force of development. Investment in the expansion of health and hygiene facilities and in general improvement of the conditions of living of the people in a society can be regarded as different forms of investment in human resources.

Increased access to quality health care services has been one of the thrust areas of the social development programmes being undertaken by the state government. In the wake of launching the policy of "Health for All" at the national level, the state has also made an intense effort to control communicable diseases like malaria, small pox, polio, cholera, TB, leprosy etc. Under the programme of Family Welfare Services, the number of sterilisation operations performed in the state during 2000-01 was 4586 as against 3238 sterilisation operations performed during 1999-2000. The number of IUD insertion performed during 2000-01 was 2480 as against 1721 during 1999-2000. Though sterilisation is the mainstay of the family welfare programmes, the spacing of births has become equally important of which spacing by oral pill and contraceptive are given more stress in the propagation of spacing methods. In addition to these, National School Health Programme has been extended to all PHC, CHC since 1993-94. The impetus of the programme is based on general health of the school going children. The programme specially covers the primary school children where medical check up is done every year. During 1998-99, 617 number of schools were visited and medical check up of 13939 students had been done. In the ensuing year of 1999-2000 and 2000-01 total number of schools visited were 214 and 200 with a number of children examined as many as 10257 and 5600 respectively. Another programme implemented in the state is children immunisation programme. Under Universal Immunisation Programme there were 13 383 numbers of infant fully immunised during 2000-01.

Presently the state government is providing health care through a network of 7 hospitals, 9 community health centres, 45 primary health centres, 13 subsidiary health centres and 351 sub-centres with a total bed strength of 1554. Supplementary nutrition programme is being implemented through the network of 21 ICDS project where 79,935 number of malnourished children (0-36 months) have benefitted during 2000-01. There were also 1341 number of Anganwadi Centres with an enrolment of 1,50,652 children in Mizoram.

Water supply and Sanitation

The provision of safe drinking water and sanitation facilities are basic necessity of life and crucial inputs in achieving the goal of "Health for All." With the launching of the Five Year Plan, the state government is envisaged to providing adequate safe drinking water and appropriate sanitation facilities to all the habitations in Mizoram. During the 9th Five Year Plan, the approved outlay for water supply and sanitation was Rs. 144.76 crores, out of which Rs. 31 crores was for rural water supply and sanitation and Rs. 93.76 crores was for urban water supply and sanitation.

The state government provides drinking water through piped water supply, rain water harvesting scheme, hand pump tube well, submersible pump and improvement of village spring sources. Sanitation facilities for rural habitations are being provided by constructing low cost sanitary latrines. At present all villages/habitations were already provided with at least one source of water supply as shown in Table 11.2.

Table 11.2
Supply of water in Mizoram

Sl. No.	Category	No. of villages covered
1	N.C.	Nil
2	P.C.	544
3	F.C.	369

Source: Socio-Economic Review Mizoram Uro-01

Note : Non-covered (NC) : village not covered with any source of drinking water
Partially Covered (PC) : Villages covered but less than 40 lpcd
Fully Covered (FC) : Villages covered with 40 lpcd or more.

Rural Development

Levels of living measured in terms of consumption expenditure of the households and individuals is one of the indicators of quality of life. While increase in average per capita income over the years suggests significant improvement in levels of living, the structural dimension of this objective is perceived in terms of the changes in the incidence of absolute poverty. The alleviation of poverty has been the central objective of development planning. Various special programmes have been in operation over the decades focussing on the poor as the target group. Some of the prominent centrally sponsored schemes implemented in Mizoram are SGSY, EAS, JGSY, PMGY. Besides, New land use policy meant to shift rural jhumias to viable schemes for permanent occupation, construction of community hall and National Programme on Improved Chulhas are being implemented. The main objectives of all these programmes have been to uplift the people living below poverty line by providing self employment through income generating activities, to provide wage employment to rural people and to create permanent assets for strengthening the rural economy. All these poverty alleviation programmes are implemented through the network of 22 Rural Development Blocks and District Rural Development Agencies (DRDA) in every districts.

Based on the sample survey data on consumer expenditure made available by National Sample Survey Organisation (NSSO) from its 55 Round Survey (July 1999-June 2000), the poverty ratio on a 30 day recall basis, the incidence of poverty expressed as a percentage of people living below poverty line has witnessed a steady decline in all the seven states. However, the ratio is relatively still higher than the national average in all the states except Mizoram in 1999-2000 (Table 11.3).

Table 11.3

Relative Poverty Ratio of North Eastern States

(per cent)

States	1973-74	1993-94	1999-2000
Arunachal Pradesh	51.93	39.35	33.47
Assam	51.21	40.86	36.09

(Contd...)

Manipur	49.96	33.78	28.54
Meghalaya	50.20	37.92	33.87
Mizoram	50.32	25.66	19.47
Nagaland	50.81	37.92	32.67
Tripura	51.00	39.01	34.44
All India	**54.88**	**38.97**	**26.10**

Poverty Ratio of Assam is used for all the States.
Source : Planning Commission.

Economic growth expressed in terms of increases in per capita income should be accompanied by a broader enhancement of human well being and quality of life. This include not only an adequate level of consumption of food and other consumer goods but also access to basic social services, especially education, health, drinking water and basic sanitation. It also includes the expansion of economic and social opportunities for all individuals and groups, reduction in disparities and a greater participation in the decision making process. The attainment of these goals not only necessitates a substantial allocation of resources but also involves an enhanced role for the government in the provision of social services, rural infrastructure, road development, etc.

In recognition of the enhanced role of government in human resource development, the government of Mizoram has increased the resource allocations for social sector components. The over all total government expenditure on social services and rural development, has increased sharply from Rs.51.45 crores in the Fifth Plan to Rs. 1775.56 crores in the Ninth Plan. As a per cent to total revenue expenditure, the social sector expenditure has increased from 29.31 per cent in the Fifth Plan to 40.24 per cent in the Ninth Plan. Growth trend and pattern of revenue expenditure are presented in Table 11.4. The table exhibits that there is a continuous and secular growth trend from the Fifth Plan to the successive Five Year Plans in education and health and family welfare. Thus, despite severe budgetary constraints being faced, the state government has enhanced allocations for the social sectors.

Table 11.4
Growth Trend of Revenue Expenditure on Social Services in Mizoram

	5th Plan	6th Plan	7th Plan	8th Plan	9th Plan
1	2	3	4	5	6
Social Services+ Rural Development	51.45 (29.31)	147.50 (34.07)	383.65 (39.45)	1033.00 (43.58)	1775.56 (40.24)
Education	22.74 (12.96)	56.96 (13.16)	134.71 (13.86)	(386.78) (16.32)	784.60 (17.78)
Health & Family Welfare	7.56 (4.31)	20.88 (4.82)	49.71 (5.11)	130.13 (5.49)	255.42 (5.79)
Water Supply, Sanitation, Housing & Urban Dev.	8.90 (5.07)	42.15 (9.74)	90.58 (9.32)	167.74 (7.08)	242.85 (5.50)
Welfare of SC/ST & Other Backward			24.07 (2.48)	98.98 (4.18)	197.63 (4.48)
Social Welfare and Nutrition	7.05 (4.02)	17.73 (4.10)	43.44 (4.47)	70.30 (2.97)	105.48 (2.39)
Others	1.37 (0.74)	3.14 (0.73)	7.64 (0.79)	19.91 (0.84)	34.59 (0.78)
Rural Development	3.83 (2.18)	6.64 (1.53)	33.50 (3.45)	159.16 (6.72)	154.99 (3.51)

Source: Statistical Handlook of Mizoram, Various Issues.
Note : Figures in Parentheses are percentage)

There has been significant progress in human development as reflected in broad indicators such as the improvements registered in educational attainments of the people, status of health, the provision of basic social infrastructure, increase in income in terms of real purchasing power for life sustenance. These three parameters are captured in the formulation of Human Development Index (HDI) by UNDP (1990). This is an attempt to evaluate the efficiency of the economy in translating the growth of income into a fairly good standard of human development. Another approach to human development which is called Gender Disparity Index (GDI) captures the position and power of female as compared to those of their male counterparts. Human Poverty Index (HPI) prepared to capture the deprivation in three dimensions of human development such as economic education and health. The proportion of population living below poverty line, who do not have access to safe drinking water, sanitation, electricity, medical care, are living in kutcha houses, illiterates and having less than 40 life expectantly at birth are incorporated in an index to measure the quality of life of the population. The position of Mizoram on Human and Poverty Indices is relatively better than the rest of the states of north east India and comparatively well in Gender Development also. The relative position of North East states is shown in Table 11.5.

Table 11.5
Relative Development Index of the North East States

States	HDI - 1991			HPI - 1991		GDI - 1991	
	Value	Rank	Modified	Value	Rank	Value	Rank
Arunachal Pradesh	0.328	29	22	49.62	30	0.776	18
Assam	0.348	26	19	48.95	27	0.575	30
Manipur	0.536	9	4	41.63	21	0.815	3
Meghalaya	0.365	24	18	49.19	28	0.807	12
Mizoram	0.548	7	3	32.2	14	0.776	
Nagaland	0.486	11	5	42.07	22	0.729	21
Tripura	0.389	22	16	44.89	24	0.531	29
India	0.381			36.36		0.676	

Source : National Development Report, 2001.

Conclusion

Judging from the preceding analysis it is evident that efforts that have been taken so far to improve quality of life, to reduce over all poverty level and to widen access to basic necessities of life have to a great extent yielded positive results. To achieve the goal of Education for All and Health for All, it is necessary to create a congenial environment that would invite a mix of public-private partnership and participation of NGOs. This will definitely improve the cost efficiency and effectiveness of these services.

In spite of all the positive results that have been exhibited by different human development indices, the ground reality shows a different picture It is found that there is a sharp difference in the living standard between the urban and the rural areas. One will find high distortion in the distribution of income. The life style of the elite class in urban North East is no less extravagant than the elites of any other state They live in imposing houses with well manicured lawns to match. Moreover these houses are beautifully equipped with all the latest hi–tech furniture and equipments. Buying the latest model of cars does not seem to cause a dent in their fat bank accounts They travel all over the world and their children are staying abroad or studying in the best schools and colleges in the country. So they are a class apart. It is therefore a fact that a handful of families control very large percentage of the state budget while on the other hand thousands or rather lakhs of families are in a state of deprivation

Basically, the North East Region is an agrarian society where the bulk of the people, about 80 per cent, depend on agriculture and allied activities. However, due to the neglect of agriculture sector, the plight of rural people has increased manifold. Problems of unemployment has become rampant among the rural youths. Because of this worsening condition, many rural people have been migrating to urban centres in search of wage-employment. The fact that the rapid growth of urbanisation is a clear indication of the stagnating situation in the rural areas. In Mizoram 49.49 per cent of the population of the state live in urban areas. Aizawl, the capital of the state alone accommodates more than 25 per cent of the state population. This trend of urbanisation is likely to continue so long the investment in rural development does not reach the people for whom the money is invested. To reduce the incidence of poverty and the pressure of unemployment, it is necessary to implement second generation reforms which promote employment growth in both agricultural and industrial sectors.

REFERENCES

Basic Statistics of North Eastern Region, 2002, Government of India, NEC, Shillong.

Bhattacharjee, R.P., Upadhaya, N.(2002) : 'Human Development in North East India', in Bimal J. Deb (ed) *Development Priorities in North East India,* Concept Publishing Company, New Delhi.

Economic Survey (2001-2002), Govt. of India, Ministry of Finance, Economic Division

Mehta, MM., 1976 : Human Resource Development Planning.

Socio-Economic Review, Mizoram, 2000-01,Directorate of Economics & Statistics, Mizoram, Aizawl.

Statistical Hand Book, Mizoram, various issues, Directorate of Economics & Statistics, Mizoram, Aizawl.

Section -III
Human Development and Well being

12

DIMENSIONS OF HUMAN RESOURCE DEVELOPMENT IN NORTH-EAST INDIA IN THE ERA OF ECONOMIC REFORMS

– *Santanu Ray*

Introduction

Human Development, a concept of about expanding peoples' choices, has perhaps been the greatest discovery of the last century in the analysis and measurement of progress. The concept is developed on the belief that people must become active agents of social change and direct beneficiaries of economic and social activities. Much quantifiable measurement of development – HDI, that redefines the wealth of nation from a holistic approach, involves three components: income, health and education, however, goes well beyond these three. The attention devoted by the new paradigm of human development is to bring the fact into the focus that people must be taken as the ends of development process rather a mere means. The concept is fundamentally about freedoms and dignity and the role of freedom in development. To enlarge peoples' choices the most critical attainments are to lead a long and healthy life; to be educated and to enjoy a decent standard of life. The capability approach argues that the goal of any public policy and action is to enlarge a person's functioning and capacity to function or expand the range of activities that a person can efficiently perform (Sen : 2005). The capability of an individual, as defined in

UNDP literature, includes the enabling opportunities given by schooling, health services etc. Additional choices include political freedom; other guaranteed human rights and various ingredients of self respect.

In post-colonial regime, there emerged a territory, commonly referred as North-East India, with a set of special features like landlockness, poor expansion of economic opportunities, immigration, ethnic turmoil, insurgency etc. Over the years, this geographical entity, endowed with many diversities in economic, political, social and cultural aspects, was bunched deliberately together into one for popular, academic as well as for administrative references. Political formalization of this bunching was completed in 1972 by the formation of North-East Council (NEC). At present it comprises of the state of Assam and the states that were curbed out from Assam at different points in time viz. Nagaland, Meghalaya and Mizoram; two former princely states of Manipur and Tripura; former North-Eastern Frontier Agency – Arunachal Pradesh. Later, the inclusion of Sikkim under NEC made the number of north eastern states to eight. A number of parallel narratives on India's north east are common in circulation. The most dominant one is about the economic deceleration of Assam since early 1980s which is primarily responsible for socio-economic unrest and ethnic turmoil of the entire region. Others praise achievements in social sector made by few small states in the region – especially Mizoram, Manipur, Nagaland and Tripura which often creates typical confusion in the literature when such achievements are taken as synonymous to human development.

II State of Human Development in NE India

The discourse of development and its measurement, which received serious attention in the latter half of the last century, discovered the holistic view that the real wealth of a nation is its people. Hence to measure the level of development of a nation the traditional indicator of per capita income should not be the sole criterion. The link between people and their living conditions must be taken into account. This approach argues that income and well-being of the people are philosophically distinct and therefore, the composite index, HDI, had been formulated by UNDP in 1990. The index takes the achievements in three attainments of a country/ region/ state/ district into consideration: income, education and health. However, the experience reveals that the attainments in other two are largely dependent on income and of course to a certain extent on the efficiency and priorities of public management to deliver health and educational services to the people at large. The selection of indicators to capture the achievements in these three aspects, however, depends upon the agency assessing the level of development. For example, to measure economic attainment of Indian states and Union Territories, Planning Commission (2002), instead of considering UNDP's 'Real Per Capita GDP adjusted for purchasing power parity', selects 'Real Per Capita Consumption Expenditure adjusted for inequality' '*to make it amenable to inter-temporal, and inter-spatial comparisons.*' In an another effort, Celliah and Shanmugam (2002), to capture same attainments, choose 'the share of non-primary sector along with the conventional per capita GDP. Chatterjee (2005) proposes an alternative index of human development taking general level as well as extent of inequality of the distribution of all attainments into account. The indicators adopted by Planning Commission (2002) to capture the achievements and setbacks in three attainments are summarized in Box 12.1.

The relative position of eight Northeastern states [computed from (Planning Commission : 2002] in the list of twenty-five Indian states during 1980s and 1990s in terms of Human Development Index (HDI); Human Poverty Index (HPI) and Gender Disparity Index (GDI) reveals altogether a mixed picture. Few unusual features are also observed in connection with these

Box 12.1 Human Development Attainment

I. ECONOMIC ATTAINMENT		
Indicator	**Maximum**	**Minimum**
1. Real Per Capita Consumption Expenditure (in Rs. / Month)	325	65
II. EDUCATIONAL ATTAINMENT		
Indicator	**Maximum**	**Minimum**
1. Literacy Rate for 7+ years of age	100	0
2. Intensity of Formal Education (adjusted for population)	7	0
III. HEALTH ATTAINMENT		
Indicators	**Maximum**	**Minimum**
1. Life Expectancy at Age 1 (in years)*	80	50
2. Infant Mortality Rate (per 1000 live births)		20

Note : Except Assam there has been no estimation so far in NE India for this indicator. Considering the direct association between life expectancy and 60+ population (relative to total population) we included the ranks of NE states in Table: 12.3.

three composite indices. The Ranks obtained by NE states in these indices are depicted in Tables 12.1 and 12.2. In 1981, Manipur was ranked second and Mizoram fourth in HDI while Arunachal Pradesh twenty-fourth among all-25 states in the country. In HPI, Mizoram and Nagaland, securing twelfth and thirteenth position in the country emerged as best and second best in the region. Arunachal Pradesh had been the worst performer in the country while Assam could manage only twenty-second position. The socio-cultural uniqueness that Manipur, Meghalaya and Nagaland inherited from their ancient past was clearly reflected in GDI ranking. These states were ranked third, eighth and eleventh respectively and were best three performers in the region. However, Assam had emerged as worst performer and Tripura was placed just before Assam.

Table -12.1 State of Human Development in NE India.

State	1981						1991					
	Rural		Urban		Combined		Rural		Urban		Combined	
	Value	Rank	Value	Rank	Value	Rank	Value	Rank	Value	Rank	Value	Rank
Arunachal Pradesh	.228	21	.419	19	.242	24	.300	21	.572	10	.328	22
Assam	.261	19	.380	23	.272	19	.326	20	.555	14	.348	19
Manipur	.440	2	.553	3	.461	2	.503	3	.618	8	.536	4
Meghalaya	.293	14	.442	16	.317	15	.332	18	.624	6	.365	18
Mizoram	.381	5	.558	2	.411	4	.464	4	.648	3	.548	3
Nagaland	.295	13	.519	5	.328	14	.442	7	.633	4	.486	5
Sikkim	.302	10	.515	7	.342	12	.398	11	.618	7	.425	12
Tripura	.264	16	.498	8	.287	18	.368	14	.551	15	.389	16
India	*.263*	-	*.442*	-	*.302*	-	*.340*	-	*.511*	-	*.381*	-
Best Performer	.491 Kerala	1	.600 Himachal **Pradesh**	1	.500 Kerala	1	.576 Kerala	1	.700 Himachal **Pradesh**	1	**.591 Kerala**	1
Worst Performer	.209 Madhya Pradesh	25	.368 Orissa	25	.237 Bihar	25	.282 Madhya Pradesh	25	.444 Uttar Pradesh	25	.308 Bihar	25

Source: Planning Commission, 2002 [Tables: 1.1, 1.2]

Table: 12.2
Ranks of NE States in Three Indices

State	1981			1991		
	HDI	HPI	GDI	HDI	HPI	GDI
Arunachal Pradesh	24	25	21	22	23	12
Assam	19	22	25	19	21	23
Manipur	2	15	3	4	15	2
Meghalaya	15	19	8	18	22	7
Mizoram	4	12	13	3	8	4
Nagaland	14	13	11	5	16	14
Sikkim	12	18	16	12	11	15
Tripura	18	16	24	16	18	22
Best Performer	Kerala	Goa	Kerala	Kerala	Kerala	Kerala
Worst Performer	Bihar		Assam	Bihar	Bihar	Biha

Source: *Planning Commission, 2002 [Tables: 1.1, 1.2, 1.3 and 1.4]*

In 1991, three neighboring states: Mizoram, Manipur and Nagaland occupied first three places in the region with national ranking of third, fourth and fifth respectively in HDI. Arunachal Pradesh improved her position from twenty-fourth in 1981 to twenty- second in 1991; however, Assam remained at nineteenth in the country. In HPI, Mizoram improved her relative position by four places (from twelfth in 1981 to eighth in 1991), Sikkim, surprisingly by seven places, Arunachal Pradesh by two and Assam by one. On the contrary, Meghalaya and Nagaland deteriorated their position relatively by three places and Tripura by two. In GDI, all states in the region except Nagaland improved significantly. Manipur improved by one point and stands second best in the country. Mizoram and Arunachal Pradesh recorded improvements each by nine points, which placed Mizoram at fourth best state in the country in gender parity. Assam's relative improvement by two points in 1991 relieves her from the position of worst performer in GDI. Nagaland deteriorated from eleventh in 1981 to fourteenth in 1991.

In national perspective, the indices of HDI and HPI are observed to be closely connected (r_R = +.801 in 1981 and r_R =

+.763 in 1991) indicating that a state with decent ranking in human development is likely to secure a fair position in human poverty ranking. However, very few exceptions in this regard occur in case of NE states. Manipur and Mizoram in 1981 and Manipur and Nagaland in 1991 were the exceptional states where the difference in HDI and HPI ranks were observed highest in the country. This indicates that the achievements in human development were unable to reach all sections proportionately. Again, the positive association between HDI and GDI; observed in case of Indian states (r_R = +.765 in 1981 and r_R = + .729 in 1991) breaks down in Meghalaya, Arunachal Pradesh (and of course in Rajasthan). The comparison of the relative positions in these two parameters for such states establishes that in 1991 their performance in gender parity go well ahead their performance in human development. In contrast, in Nagaland the fifth position in HDI coincides with fourteenth position in GDI, which indicates clearly that level of human development is not engendered - failing to widen the choices and opportunities of women as compared to their male counterpart.

A special feature in this regard is note worthy – Rural-Urban Disparity in the level of human development. While during 1980's the gap in national level narrowed down marginally, the same widened significantly in all the states in the region excepting Tripura and Nagaland. This feature is summarized in Fig.12.1. In 1981, the disparity in Tripura, Nagaland, Sikkim and Arunachal Pradesh had been estimated higher than Indian average. In 1991 states of Meghalaya, Assam and Mizoram were included in the list. Interestingly, in 1991 values of HDI in urban areas of all NE states were above national urban average. Moreover, the HDI values in urban Mizoram and Manipur during 1981 and in urban Mizoram in 1991 were recorded even higher than that of Kerala.

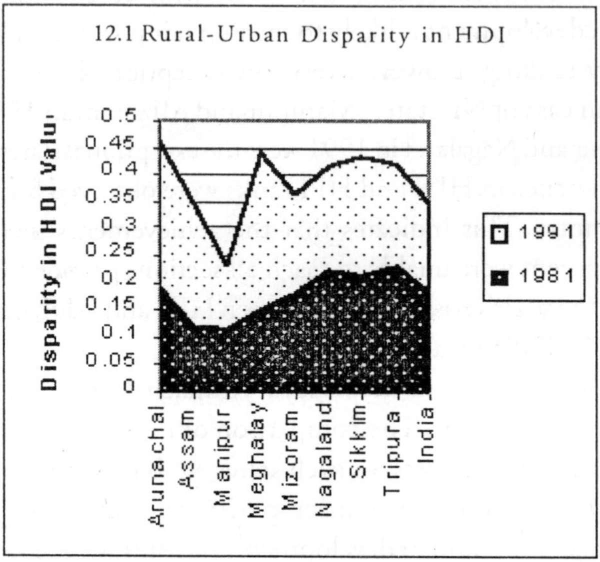

The achievements in absolute value of human development index and corresponding rank for each NE state in 1991, as depicted in Table 12.3, reveal a very different story for each state. We shall compare the HDI ranking of each state to their ranks in three attainments. Mizoram - the best performer in the region could achieve the status of third best state in the country mainly due to the spectacular performances in economic and educational attainments. The state ranks first (among all-25 Indian states) in Real Per Capita Consumption Expenditure and second in Literacy Rate (for 7+ age group) while other indicators are significantly below the overall HDI position. Manipur occupies second position in Infant Mortality Rate and fifth in Intensity of Formal Education as compared to her fourth best position in HDI. Nagaland, the fifth state in the country in terms of human development, achieves this standard on the strength of consumption expenditure and to some extent on literacy rate. However, the ranks of Sikkim in almost all indicators are found to be at per to her HDI position. Decent level of consumption expenditure and literacy rate in Tripura fails to achieve a decent level of overall HDI position mainly due to the poor performances in Intensity of Formal Education.

Table: 12.3
Ranks in Attainment - Indicators (NE States)

HDI								
State	Rank	Rank in Economic Indicator RPCCE?	Attainments Educational Indicators 7+ LR	IFE	EL at 1	1991 Health Indicators % *of 60+ Pop.*		IMR
		α	β	χ	δ	ε		ϕ
		1993-94	1991	1993 (adj)	1993 (non-adj)	1991-95	*1991*	1991
Arunachal Pradesh	22	15	22	15	23	NE	*25*	20
Assam	19	19	16	16	17	15	*19*	21
Manipur	4	9	10	5	10	NE	*17.5*	2
Meghalaya	18	5	17	18	25	NE	*23*	16
Mizoram	3	1	2	8	20	NE	*21*	6
Nagaland	5	2	7	24	22	NE	*20*	3.5
Sikkim	12	13	13	13	16	NE	*22*	9
Tripura	16	8	9	23	15	NE	*8*	17.5
Best Performer	Kerala	Mizoram	Kerala	Goa	Goa	Kerala	*Kerala H.P.*	Kerala
Worst Performer	Bihar	Bihar	Bihar	Bihar	Meghalaya	Assam	*A.P.*	M.P

Notes: α: Real per capita Consumption Expenditure (Rs/month), β: Literacy Rate for 7+ years of age, χ: Intensity of Formal Education (adjusted for population) & (non-adjusted), δ: Life Expectancy at Age 1 (in years), ε: Percent of 60+ populations to total population, ϕ: Infant Mortality Rate (per 1000 live births)

In Meghalaya high consumption level coincides with poor performance in all other indicators. Assam, the most populous state in the region which plays a crucial role in determining the regional average in all aspects, is placed on nineteenth position due to almost parallel performances in all attainments. Arunachal Pradesh, the worst performer in north-east, repeats the story of Assam.

Table: 12.4 Relative Economic Features of NE States during 1990-91

(Figures in rupees)

State	Gross State Domestic Product Per Capita		Gross Central Devolution Per Capita		Productivity*	
	Relative Value	Rank	Relative Value	Rank	Relative Value	Rank
Arunachal Pradesh	104.32	10	829.35	2	26.67	24
Assam	87.01	19	178.31	11	83.57	13
Manipur	80.62	21	460.44	5	38.87	23
Meghalaya	103.48	11	375.31	9	65.72	16
Mizoram	101.75	13	1051.60	1	07.68	25
Nagaland	114.56	6	753.41	3	44.14	21
Sikkim	108.30	9	673.61	4	46.92	20
Tripura	84.86	20	385.35	7	66.29	15
NE States	89.72	-	288	-	71.73	-
All States	100	-	100	-	100	-
Best Performer/Recipient	Goa 206.19	1	Mizoram 1051.60	1	Haryana 202.26	1
Worst Performer/Recipient	Bihar 58.40	25	Karnataka 68.28	25	Mizoram 07.68	25

Source: *Computed by Author from EPW Research Foundation (2004) & Census1991*

Table: 12.5 Ranks of NE States in Economic Indicators

States	Ranks in Economic Features				
	Agriculture	Industry	Infrastructure	Social Sector	Overall
Arunachal Pradesh	22	21	25	15	25
Assam	15	16	23	22	22
Manipur	10	22	21	14	17
Meghalaya	19	20	15	23	23
Mizoram	25	25	20	11	24
Nagaland	23	18	16	17	21
Sikkim	13	24	19	12	16
Tripura	14	19	22	16	20
Best Performer	**Punjab**	**Gujarat**	**Punjab**	**Maharasthra**	**Punjab**
Worst Performer	Mizoram	Mizoram	Arunachal Pradesh	Jammu & Kashmir	Arunachal Pradesh

Source: *Goswami. H & J.K. Gogoi (2004)*

Table: 12.6 Improvement (-) / Deterioration (+) of Gini Ratios for Per Capita Consumption Expenditure during 1990s (NE States)

States	Rural		Urban	
	Change	Rank	Change	Rank
Arunachal Pradesh	-.008	18	+.023	21
Assam	+.025	24	+.026	22
Manipur	+.043	25	+.063	24.5
Meghalaya	-.122	1	-.034	3
Mizoram	+.023	23	+.063	24.5
Nagaland	+.002	21	+.011	18
Sikkim	+.014	22	+.007	16
Tripura	-.047	5	+.015	20
India	-.024	-	+.001	-
Highest Improvement	Meghalaya	1	Himachal Pradesh	1
Worst Deterioration	Manipur	25	Mizoram & Manipur	24.5 24.5

Source: Planning Commission, 2002 [Table: 2.3]

III Economic and Human Development: Linkage and Causality

The principle underpinning human capital theory is the belief that the peoples' learning capacities are of comparable value to other resources involved in production of goods and services (Lucas : 1990). Human resource like any other resource, if utilized effectively, gives a return what is profitable for the individual who produces it as well for the society at large in which s/he belongs. The theory establishes through empirical studies the gains of education and training as a form of investment in human resources. People are considered as a form of capital for development. Similarly, economic growth theory emphasizes on the role of quality of the factors of production in determining the rate of growth of an economy. The revolution that has taken place in growth theory and growth models in last few decades has been basically the rediscovery of the fact that higher human capital formation leads to a higher growth of output and total factor productivity. The journey from Solow-Swan of neoclassical school to Easterly-Levine-Rebelo as well as Lucas-Romar of endogenous growth theory enriches our wisdom with a set of stylized facts which reestablishes the importance of savings in the formation of wealth of nations. Studies by Mankiw, Romar and Weil document the high association between the educational attainment of labour force and total factor productivity. More recent addition in the literature by Schaper (2003) and Muysken (2003) reveal that education and health policiės of the economy affect both income distribution and growth rate. The world-wide wave of new emphasis that UNDP places on human capabilities is no way limited to the mere development of social sector. It is argued categorically in UNDP literature that human development and economic growth are closely connected. There are evidences which establish that economic growth alone may not be able to benefit everyone in the society. However, for long-run sustainable welfare of the people a meaningful and uninterrupted economic growth has been inevitable – a most important means in this regard. A much wider and more inclusive perspective of development has been conceptualized in the label of human development. The ultimate purpose perhaps is to monitor whether growth of an economy is being translated into improvements of people's lives and if so, in what extent. The concept of human development is not a focus on social issues at the expense of economic issues. The holistic doctrine of development prescribes a form of investment in basic health and nutrition, in literacy and education on basic economic assumption that '*healthy and educated people can, through productive employment, contribute more to economic growth*' UNDP (1992). Sustainable human development paradigm intends '*to address both intragenerational and intergenerational equity – enabling all generations, present and future to make the best use of their potential capabilities*' UNDP (1994). The paradigm regards economic growth as a means - not an end; concerns about the life opportunities of future generations and respects the natural systems on which all lives of present and future generations depend.

In national level studies the causality between economic and human development have been attempted to establish in both ways. Few Scholars find that economic growth determines the level of human development, however, others argue for reverse causality. Dholakia (2003) finds that human development indicators positively influence income with a lag of about eight years, whereas, income per capita affects the other within two years. There exists argument neither in human capital or growth theory nor in UNDP literature which recognizes the human development indicators as independent events - not linked to economic progress. However, new development paradigm has been emphasizing the role of growth in human development. Achievements in human development indicators without corresponding achievements in economic front often face the question of sustainability. What is of more concern is that such achievements remain as mere success of social sector – fails miserably to fulfill broader goal of human development. The studies, undertaken by national mainstream scholars to establish the causal relationship between economic and human development or to examine regional disparities in post-reform period, mostly concentrate on '*major states*'. Except Assam all northeastern states are conventionally excluded for the simple reason that '*they are too small to reflect the general economic behaviour of states of India*' (Bhattacharya and Saktivel : 2004). Other serious problem which comes on the way is that lack of authentic time series data for these states. Consequently, issues related to NE states mostly remain unaddressed and it appears that there have been no such concerns that need to be examined on national perspective.

The studies, undertaken by the scholars of the region, mostly concentrate on the eight states of the region. Among very few that attempted to analyse the performance of NE states in national perspective, Bezbaruah and Dutta (2004) is important. The paper, adopting an alternative line of analysis, compared relative per capita income of NE states with national average and concluded that as time passed the economic indicators show a clear downward trend for the region as a whole and few states in particular. Goswami and Gogoi (2004) rank all 25 Indian states on the basis of an indicator, called *overall composite index of development*. Achievements of the states in economic field are measured in their work - not by the conventional per capita state income but through a set of selected indicators in four sectors: agriculture, industry, infrastructure and social sector. The relative position assigned to NE states in four sectors as well as in *overall composite index of development* are briefly summarized in Table: 12.5. These ranks are adopted to examine the economic-human development trade-off in northeast India in Fig.12.2.

Economists have different opinions to consider per capita income as an indicator of economic performance. The intention of the chapter paper is altogether different from taking part into that debate. However, there is a serious problem to accept GSDP

Fig. 12.2 : Economic-Human Development Trade–off in Indian States

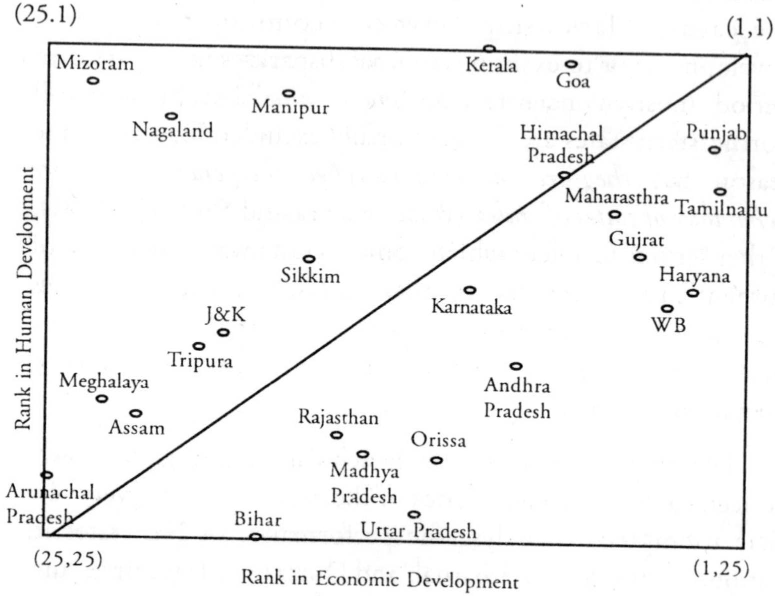

as an economic indicator in case of NE states. Of the two distinct components of state income, namely, that originating within the state, and receiving as Gross Central Devolution (GCD), it is the former that mainly determines the state income in most of the Indian states. The latter comprises below 9 per cent of GSDP during the fiscal year 1990-91 in all-state average. Not surprisingly, in NE region the significance of gross central devolution which consists of shares in central taxes, grants, loans etc had been above 28 per cent. This is due to the fact that the biggest economy in the region – Assam received 18 per cent of her GSDP which pulled down the regional average significantly. The gross central devolution relative to GSDP in small states of the region ranges from 89 percent in Mizoram to 32 per cent in Meghalaya. What is noteworthy here is that the gross central devolution is likely to increase the state income and in turn the disposable income, however, is not able to enlarge the economic opportunity of the people. At least this can not be accepted as an indicator of economic attainment. An indicator in this regard should reflect the productive capacity and productive efficiency of the resources employed within a state. The indicator capturing economic attainment should suit conceptually to the note '*...the income of a person can tell us a good deal about her ability to do things that she has reason to value*' (Anand and Sen : 2000).

Total factor productivity, commonly termed as *residual factor* and identified as contribution of *human capital* in production function, would have been the right indicator. Given the scope of this chapter and shortcomings of available data-base of the region we simply attempt to measure productivity - the productive capacity of an individual, captured by the size of average return in a given year, in each Indian state. This measure reflects the level of opportunity that is being offered to a person by the state for her/his efficient functioning. Productivity in this regard is defined as the component of GSDP originated within the state divided by the total strength of the labour force engaged where marginal workers are assigned weights exactly half of main workers i.e. [GSDP – GCD] / [Main + ½ Marginal workers]. The Indian states, if ranked according to their productivity in 1990-91 (as depicted in Table: 12.4.), Mizoram, Arunachal Pradesh and Manipur are placed in last three positions while Nagaland and Sikkim are in twenty-first and twentieth position. The best performer in the region has been Assam which occupies thirteenth position in the country. When the poorest state in the country – Bihar scores above 65 per cent relative to all-state average, the performances of Mizoram, Arunachal Pradesh and Manipur are found as poor as 8 per cent, 27 per cent and 39 per cent respectively. The relative positions of NE states in per capita central devolution are very high – first five positions in the country are well secured by Mizoram, Arunachal Pradesh, Nagaland, Sikkim and Manipur. Tripura, Meghalaya and Assam are in seventh, ninth and eleventh position respectively. On the contrary, Bihar and Orissa – twentieth and thirteenth recipients of central assistance - received 81 per cent and 123 per cent relative to all-state average. The same stands at 1052 per cent for Mizoram, 829 per cent for Arunachal Pradesh and 753 per cent for Nagaland. This unprecedented incidence of central devolution is reflected clearly in per capita consumption expenditure of NE states which has been projected as the sole indicator of economic attainment in Planning Commission (2002). In no way we suggest any caution to existing rate of central assistance to these states. The problem arises precisely to accept such feature as tantamount to wider level of economic opportunity in a comparative study. For instance, if the states like Bihar and Orissa would have been blessed by Finance Commission at a rate, similar to that of Mizoram, Arunachal Pradesh or Nagaland, the level of consumption expenditure, literacy etc which determine the absolute value of HDI could be very different from present level.

IV A Diagrammatic Representation

The ranks of all 25 Indian states in overall economic development, if compared to their corresponding ranks in human development index, exibit a weak association (r_R = +.325). However, exclusion of eight NE states improves the coefficient significantly (r_R = +.712). This indicates clearly that positive association between two developmental aspects breaks down in the case of NE states due to huge differences between their ranks in economic and human development. The relative positions of each state in these two parameters are plotted in Fig. 12.2 where economic development and human development ranks are depicted in horizontal and vertical axes respectively. The origin (25,25) denotes the case of hypothetical state that ranks worst in both. Similarly, the opposite corner (1,1) represents the state that stands best in both. However, the corners (1,25) and (25,1) denote the situations when the state stands best in one and worst in other. In our diagram four quadrants namely HH, LH, LL, and HL can be categorized. Indian states are mostly scattered in HH and LL quadrants indicating that a state attains a decent rank in either of the two assures likelihood to secure a decent position in other. Instead ranks in overall economic development, productivity is used as an indicator of economic development, no change in terms of quadrants is observed in case of NE states. However, few minor shifts from HL to LL and LL to HL are noted for Andhra Pradesh, Orissa and Rajasthan and Uttar Pradesh respectively. Four NE states belong to LH while other four in LL in both occasions as in Box: 12.2. The states namely Meghalaya, Assam and Arunachal Pradesh are placed in LL indicating a poor rank in Human development is coupled with unsatisfactory rank in economic opportunity. Other four states in the region Mizoram, Nagaland, Manipur and Sikkim have emerged in both occasions as the case of decent rank in human development coinciding with very poor position in economic opportunity.

Further extension of this diagrammatic analysis would clear the dimension of human development in northeastern states. Each point on the chord connecting the corners (1,1) and (25,25) signifies that the state has emerged with same rank in both. The achievements in economic front are translated into an appropriate achievement in human development. In other words, the expansion of capabilities is properly accomplished with parallel expansion of opportunities. Further away the state is from this chord of balanced development denotes the higher level of imbalance between human and economic development. The states lying below this line imply the common and vividly discussed feature of national developmental experience – the economic progress failed to get translated into a parallel level of capability building. Thirteen states in the country belong to this category. On the contrary, the position of any state above the line of balance indicates a different aspect of development debacle: achievements in human development are not accomplished with economic opportunities. At least eleven states, as in Figure: 12.2, have been sufferer (of course in different extents) of such phenomenon. All northeastern states suffer from this feature of lopsided development syndrome. Other states

Box.12.2: Classification of Indian States

LH	HH
Mizoram, Nagaland, Manipur, Sikkim	Kerala, Goa, Punjab, Himachal Pradesh,Tamilnadu, Karnataka, Maharasthra,Haryana, Gujrat,
LL	**HL**
J & K, Tripura, Meghalaya, Assam, Arunachal Pradesh, Rajasthan, Madhya Pradesh, Uttar Pradesh, Bihar	West Bengal, Andhra Pradesh Orissa

V Observations and Conclusion

Despite sufficient national and international acclaim, questions are regularly raised against the framework of so-called *Kerala Model* which emphasized the role of planned public investment in social sector without concerning much on economic front. Few social indicators, as reported in media, do not establish that social achievements could accomplish at large. The pessimism about sustainability of Kerala's development debacle, expressed in Kannan (1990) and also in Jeromi (2003), somehow turns into a very recent optimistic note in Kannan (2005). However, scant attention has been paid to the lopsided development achievements in northeastern states. Huge public spending in these states come from certain compulsions what is basically different from that of Kerala. In these states that suffer from acute syndrome of unaccomplished capability, the state income, in fact, is largely determined by public expenditure. The poor economic base mainly due to inadequate economic activities compels the state governments to incur huge expenditure either by means of central assistance or by borrowings. This practice in turn deteriorates the fiscal health of the state. Moreover, public-spending-led economic structure has its typical consequences on society and governance.

The present policy-frame in each state of the region unduly emphasizes the role of elitist-state-arrangements which in turn make the development process highly exclusionary – a perverse pattern of economic activities, characterized by anti people features of excluding and concentrating. Ethnicity based political culture has often been used in different extent as powerful means to deprive people keeping them away from new opportunities. The elite domination in economic opportunities and political decisions plays a crucial role not only to control market mechanism – also to decide the matters that shape the life of general people. Regrettably, the strategy for the expansion of choices and opportunities in northeast India heads neither towards the goal of pro-*poor-growth,* advocated in mainstream World Bank Development literature nor similar to *people-centric-development* orientation, dreamt by the proponents of Alternative Development Approach.

The goal of any analysis of economic progress can not be anything other than the improvement of the condition of the people at large. In addition, human development is no way an event – rather a process that requires set of commitments from all participants of *institutional matrix.* Recently attention has been paid on the role of human development in economic performance. Meanwhile, increased emphasis is now being placed on understanding process that links economic growth, social sector development, reduction of poverty, building of capabilities and human development.

An earlier generation of development specialists and policy-makers recognized the importance of free flow of funds for all these developmental needs. Insurgency as well as violent protests by civil agitators mostly on ethnic line in different parts of the region since sixties mounted pressure on Finance Commission and other Constitutional bodies to be liberal enough in releasing funds to the region as a whole and few small states in particular. Funding agencies have been liberalizing relevant formula for NE states even in post-reform years without questioning accountability that often threatens the development itself. Several bodies are formed in last few decades on goals for removing anomalies in administrative, macroeconomic and mesoeconomic fields by which the entire region is afflicted with. Subsequently, all state governments have declared active support for these goals but when the question of implementation comes, they are conventionly forgotten. The situation resembles the age-old story about the naked king, sitting shamelessly in regular assembly and being overlooked by the puppets who are hesitant to point out the reality and trying to behave in a manner that everything is perfectly normal. The unprivileged mass - irrespective of state, community, ethnicity or religion - have been helplessly looking for the innocent lad to arrive into the assembly and courageously to point out – *King! You are naked...* Let all hope by that time it would not be too late........

REFERENCES

Anand, S & A.Sen (2000): *'The Income Component of Human Development Approach'* Journal of Human Development - an alternative approach 1(1) Feb 2000

Bezbaruah, M.P and M.K.Dutta (2004): *'Development Experience and Perspective in the North-Eastern Region'* Seminar Paper Presented in the National Seminar on Social Change in NE, April 28-30, Guwahati

Bhattachaya, B.B & S. Sakthivel (2004): *'Regional Growth and Disparity in India –Comparison of Pre and Post-Reform Decades'* Economic and Political Weekly 39(10) March 6, 2004.

Celliah, R.J & K.P. Shammugam (2002): *'Some Aspects of Inter-District Disparities in Tamil Nadu'* in Pandit. V et.al. edited 'Data, Models and Policies' – Proceedings of the 38th Annual Conference of the Indian Econometric Society.

Chatterjee, S.K (2005): *'Measurement of Human Development; An alternative approach'* Journal of Human Development - an alternative approach 6(1) March 2005

Dholakia, R.H (2003): *'Regional Disparity in Economic and Human Development in India'* Economic and Political Weekly 38(40) September 27, 2003

Easterly, W & R. Levine (1997) : *'Africa's Growth Tragedy : Policies and Ethnic Divisions'* Quarterly Journal of Economics 112, November 1997.

EPW Research Foundation (2004) : 'Finances of State Governments' Economic and Political Weekly 39(18 & 19) May 1& 8, 2004.

Goswami, H & J.K. Gogoi (2004) : *Interstate Disparities in Economic Development – With Special Reference to North Eastern States* Seminar Paper Presented in The Workshop on Quantitative Analysis in Economics March 8-13 2004 Shillong.

Jeromi, P.D (2003): *'What ails Kerala's Economy: A Sectoral Exploration'* Economic and Political Weekly 38(16) April 19, 2003

Kannan, K.P (1990): *'Kerala Economy at the Crossroad?'* Economic and Political Weekly 25(35&36) September1, 1990

Kannan, K.P (2005): *Kerala's Turnaround in Growth – Role of Social Development, Remittences and Reform'* Economic and Political Weekly 40(6) Feb.5, 2005

Lucas, R.E (1990) : *'Why Doesn't Capital flow from Rich to Poor Countries?'* American Economic Review: Paper and Proceedings 1990

Muysken, J *et.al* (2003) : *'Health, Labour Productivity and Growth'* in Hagemann. H & S. Seiter edited 'Growth Model and Growth Policy, Routledge, London

Planning Commission (2002) : *'National Human Development Report 2001'* Government of India

Ray, Santanu (2003): 'Economic Sustainability and Structural Transformation in Mizoram' in Das. G edited *Structural Change and Strategy of Development* Akansha Publishing House, New Delhi

Sachs, I (2004) : *'From the Poverty Trap to Inclusive Development in LDCs'* Economic and Political Weekly 39(18) May 1, 2004.

Schaper, C (2003) : *'Growth and Distribution Effects of Education Policy in an Endogenous Growth Model with Human Capital Accumulation'* in Hagemann. H & S. Seiter edited 'Growth Model and Growth Policy, Routledge, London.

Sen, A (2005): *'Human Rights and Human Capabilities'* Journal of Human Development - an alternative approach 6(2) July 2005

UNDP (1990) : *Human Development Report 1990* Oxford University Press.

UNDP (1992) : *Human Development Report 1992* Oxford University Press.

UNDP (1994) : *Human Development Report 1994* Oxford University Press.

UNDP (2002) : *'Avoiding the Dependency Trap: Roma Human Development Report – Challenges and Opportunities'* http://www.roma.undp.sk/right_bar.php.

UNDP (2004) : *Human Development Report 2004* Oxford University Press.

UNDP (2005) : *Human Development Report.* http://www.undp.org.in/Hdr2005

·13

LEVELS OF HUMAN DEVELOPMENT: A CASE STUDY WITH SPECIAL REFERENCE TO ASSAM

– *Padmalochan Hazarika*

Introduction

While economic growth relates to only one aspect of human life - the economic aspect, the term 'human development' embraces factors like political, cultural and social besides the economic factors. Human development is the end while economic growth is only a means to this end. The growth of an economy expressed in terms of gross national product (GNP) or the product per capita does not reflect the qualitative dimensions in the development process. Mahbub ul Haq (1971) a leading Pakistani economist has aptly remarked, "the problem of development must be defined as a selective attack on the worst forms of poverty. Development goals must be defined in terms of progressive reduction and eventual elimination of malnutrition, disease, illiteracy, unemployment and inequalities. We were taught to take care of our GNP because it would take care of poverty. Let us reverse this and take care of poverty because it will take care of GNP. In other words, let us worry about the content of GNP even more than its rate of increase."

Although human development is indeed the 'end' of all activities yet in view of the various dimensions associated with it, its measurement is not an easy task. The search for a comprehensive measure led to the definition and formulation of Human Development Index (HDI) by the UNDP in its first Human Development Report (HDR). Such an index certainly cannot incorporate the multipharious dimensions of human development yet it is superior to a long list of indicators combined with a qualitative discussion. HDI does not replace GNP but adds considerably to an understanding of the real position of a society in terms of some other vital aspects like education, health and nutrition.

The problem under Study

In this chapter we attempt to make a study relating to disparities in human development among the 23 districts of Assam on the basis of a select list of indicators of human development.

Sources of information

The study is based entirely on the secondary sources of information. Relevant data relating to the select indicators are obtained from Statistical Hand Book of Assam, 2002 and Economic Survey of Assam, 2003-2004.

Selection of indicator and methodology of study

The following indicators are taken for studying inter-district disparities in human development in Assam :

X_1 = Percentage of Literacy, X_2 = No. of primary and middle schools per 10,000 population, X_3 = No. of high school per 10,000 population, X_4 = No. of colleges per lakh population, X_5 = No. of hospitals, dispensaries per lakh population, X_6 = Infant mortality per one thousand birth, X_7 = Percentage of habitations providing with drinking water facilities, X_8 = Per Capita Gross district domestic product (in rupees) at current price, 1994-95 price.

The methodology of our study is based on the construction of a composite index on the basis of the chosen indicators of development. Most of the 'regional disparity' studies made in our country and based on three methods of constructing a composite index. They are (i) Equal Weightage Index Method or Indexing Method (ii) Ranking Method and (iii) Method of Principal Component Analysis. There is another method of construction of a composite index known as 'Deprivation Method' which gives a Human development Index (HDI). The search for a comprehensive measure that could capture the various dimensions of human development led to the definition and formulation of this index by the United Nations Development Programme (UNDP) in its Human Development Report (HDR) published in 1990. One minus deprivation index is the human development index. We have calculated the HDI's for various districts from their corresponding deprivation indices. The following three steps are involved in the construction of HDI:

In the first step, a measure of deprivation that a district suffers with respect to all the chosen indicators is obtained in terms of a formula as below :-

$$I_{ij} = \frac{\underset{j}{Max}_{ij} - X_{ij}}{\underset{j}{Max}_{ij} - \underset{j}{Min}_{ij}} \quad ....(1)$$

where I_{ij} indicates the deprivation indicator for the jth district with respect to the ith variable (indicator) and X_{ij} indicates the value of the ith indicator with respect to the jth district. However, the formula for measuring deprivation in terms of an indicator is used whenever a higher value of the indicator indicates a lesser deprivation (or higher development) in terms of the indicator. For example, this formula is used to measure deprivation in terms of percentage of literacy (X_2). If the higher value of an indicator implies higher deprivation (or lesser development) as in case of infant mortality per one thousand birth (X_6) then the formula will be as below :

$$I_{ij} = \frac{\overset{Max_{ij}}{X_{ij}} - J}{\underset{j}{Max_{ij}} - \underset{j}{Min_{ij}}} \ldots\ldots\ldots\ldots(2)$$

The deprivation index places a district in the range of zero to one.

In the second step, an average deprivation indicator (I) pertaining to each district is computed by the following formula.

$$I_{ij} = \frac{\sum_{i=1}^{n} I_{ij}}{n}$$

where n is the total no. of indicators of the percentages in respect of all the eight selected indicators. In the third step, the human development index for the jth district L = 1,2, 3, ...n is calculated by using the following formula:
(HDI) = 1 –L.,j=1,2, 3,....................n.

A district for which the HDI score lies between 0.8 and 1 (including both the values) is termed as developed. If the score point lies between 0.5 land 0.8 (including 0.5, but excluding 0.8) then the district is termed as moderately developed and if the score point is below 0.5 then the district is termed as less developed or backward.

We have also used Equal Weightage Index Method or Indexing Method to study the district level disparities in Human Development in Assam. For this we have expressed the values of all the districts relating to each indicator as percent of the corresponding state value. The sum of the indicators of a district divided by 8 gives the average HDI for the district. Since Assam is considered to be backward in terms of economic as well as human development, hence the districts whose average HDI values are greater than 100 (being the average HDI value for the state of Assam) are taken as relatively developed and others as backward.

Estimation of development indices and analysis

The data relating to the select eight human development indicators are displayed in Table 13.1. The HDI values for various districts of Assam have been estimated by Deprivation Method and tabulated (Table 13.2) and the values of HDI for the districts have also been estimated by Indexing Method and have been displayed in Table 13.3.

Table – 13.1

Assam : Human Development Indicators

Sl. No.	District	X_1	X_2	X_3	X_4	X_5	X_6	X_7	X_8
1.	Dhubri	38.31	11.95	0.90	0.15	0.37	128	63.8	5875
2.	Kokrajhar	40.57	11.97	0.76	0.24	0.71	78	57.3	5892
3.	Bongaigaon	49.06	11.70	1.08	0.24	0.64	122	52.9	6666
4.	Goalpara	46.80	13.45	1.27	0.89	0.37	106	48.3	5837
5.	Barpeta	43.24	9.49	1.62	0.93	0.43	101	40.9	6534
6.	Nalbari	55.95	9.75	1.56	0.59	0.75	96	66.2	5978
7.	Kamrup	65.04	7.27	1.24	0.54	0.52	77	56.6	8758
8.	Darrang	42.00	11.00	1.10	0.76	0.49	111	52.6	4740
9.	Sonitpur	48.14	9.41	1.04	0.21	0.44	77	70.1	6031
10.	Lakhimpur	58.96	18.16	2.67	0.53	0.48	112	64.7	7208
11.	Dhemaji	53.84	19.42	1.56	0.62	0.41	114	62.6	6191
12.	Marigoan	47.99	16.77	1.37	0.31	0.37	88	58.9	8062
13	Nagaon	54.77	14.48	0.94	0.26	0.51	97	59.1	9998
14	Golaghat	58.54	11.01	1.47	0.72	0.53	61	60.1	6955
15	Jorhat	65.51	10.59	2.31	1.95	0.62	47	69.2	6496
16	Sibsagar	64.46	10.57	1.65	0.66	0.47	57	48.4	9940
17	Dibrugarh	58.32	12.15	1.12	0.38	0.33	51	53.4	5991
18	Tinsukia	50.28	9.85	0.69	0.20	0.32	73	65.8	5282
19	Karbi	45.75	14.22	0.98	0.30	0.81	70	53.4	6675
20	Anglong	57.76	33.75	0.99	0.66	0.99	10-	65.8	5813
21	N.C.Hills	54.71	11.55	0.58	0.50	0.42	11	51.9	6909
22	Karimganj	53.07	10.51	0.62	0.50	0.22	9-	53.4	5922
23	Hailakandi	59.19	9.12	0.95	0.49	0.32	9-	48.1	14060
24	Cachar	52.89	10.86	1.23	0.50	0.48	9-	58.40	6816
	Assam	(100)	(100)	(100)	(100)	(100)	(100)	(100)	(100)

Data source : Statistical Hand Book of Assam, 2002; Economic Survey of Assam, 2003-04

From the HDI column of Table 13.2, we find that none of the districts of Assam can be termed developed as far as human development is concerned, as for none of the districts the HDI value lies between 0.8 and 1 (inclusive of both the values). The

HDI values for the districts of Jorhat, N. C. Hills, Sibsagar and Lakhimpur are 0.707, 0.547, 0.509 and 0.500 respectively and these districts can be termed moderately developed as the HDI values of these districts lie between 0.5 and 0.8 (including 0.5 but excluding 0.8). And these districts rank first, second, third and fourth respectively. For all other 19 districts the HDI values are below 0.5 and hence these districts are termed backward in terms of human development.

The Indexing method (Table 13.3) reveals that the districts of Jorhat, N.C.Hills, Lakhimpur and Sibsagar along with other 10 districts are relatively developed (RD) as the average index of each of these districts is above the state average index. The relatively developed districts of Jorhat, N.C.Hills, Lakhimpur and Sibsagar rank respectively first, second, third and fourth.

We find that both the methods rank Jorhat and N.C.Hills in the first and the second positions, while Deprivation Method places Sibsagar and Lakhimpur in the third and the fourth positions respectively, the Indexing method places these districts in the reverse order i.e., in the fourth and the third positions respectively. Since Deprivation Method gives an absolute measure of development and Indexing Method gives a relative measure hence we can say with high degree of confidence that only four districts, namely Jorhat, N. C. Hills, Sibsagar and Lakhimpur are developed to some extent or moderately developed and the remaining nineteen districts are all backward as far *as* human development in concerned. A district which is relatively developed to Assam (which is known *as* a backward or less developed state in the country) may not be even moderately developed in true sense of the term.

Epilogue

Although attaining of complete balanced regional human development may ever remain as a dream only yet unrelented efforts on the part of the planning authorities and those who are in charge of executing the various plans and programmes will go a long way in wiping out disparities in human development to a significant extent.

Table – 13.2
Human Development Indices in Districts of Assam
(By Deprivation Method)

Sl. No.	District	X_1	X_2	X_3	X_4	X_5	X_6	X_7	X_8	Total	Average Depri-vation Index	HDI	Status
1.	Dhubri	1.00	0.82	0.85	1.00	0.81	1.00	0.22	0.88	6.65	0.823	0.117	B
2.	Kokrajhar	0.92	0.82	0.91	0.95	0.36	0.38	0.18	0.88	5.40	0.675	0.325	B
3.	Bongaigaon	0.60	0.83	0.75	0.95	0.45	0.93	0.59	0.77	5.88	0.735	0.265	B
4	Goalpara	0.69	0.77	0.67	0.59	0.81	0.73	0.75	0.88	5.89	0.36	0.264	B
5	Barpeta	0.82	0.92	0.50	0.57	0.72	0.67	1.00	0.81	6.01	0.751	0.249	B
6	Nalbaru	0.35	0.91	0.53	0.76	0.31	0.60	0.13	0.87	4.46	0.558	0.442	B
7	Kamrup	0.02	1.00	0.68	0.78	0.61	0.37	0.46	0.67	4.49	0.561	0.439	B
8.	Darrang	0.86	0.86	0.75	0.66	0.65	0.79	0.26	1.00	5.83	0.729	0.271	B
9	Sonitpur	0.64	0.92	0.78	0.97	0.71	0.37	0.00	0.86	5.52	0.656	0.344	B
10	Lakhimpur	0.24	0.59	0.00	0.79	0.66	0.80	0.18	0.74	4.00	0.500	0.500	MD (4)
11	Dhemaji	0.43	0.54	0.53	0.74	0.75	0.83	0.26	0.84	4.92	0.615	0.349	B
12	Marigaon	0.64	0.64	0.62	0.91	0.81	0.51	0.38	0.64	5.15	0.644	0.356	B
13	Nagaon	0.40	0.73	0.83	0.94	0.62	0.62	0.38	0.44	4.96	0.620	0.380	B
14	Golaghat	0.26	0.86	0.86	0.68	0.60	0.17	0.35	0.76	4.25	0.531	0.469	B

(Contd.)

Sl. No.	District	X_1	X_2	X_3	X_4	X_5	X_6	X_7	X_8	Total	Average Depri-vation Index	HDI	Status
15	Jorhat	0.00	0.86	0.17	0.00	0.48	0.00	0.03	0.81	2.35	0.293	0.707	MD(1)
16	Sibsagar	0.40	0.88	0.49	0.72	0.71	0.35	0.30	0.44	3.93	0.491	0.509	MD(3)
17	Dibrugarh	0.26	0.82	0.75	0.87	0.86	0.05	0.76	0.87	5.24	0.655	0.345	B
18	Tinsukia	0.56	0.90	0.95	0.97	0.87	0.32	0.74	0.94	6.25	0.781	0.219	B
19	Kari Anglong	0.73	0.74.	0.81	0.92	0.23	0.36	0.57	0.79	5.515	0.644	0.356	B
20	N.C.Hill	0.29	0.00	0.80	0.72	0.00	0.75	0.18	0.88	3.62	0.453	0.547	MD(2)
21	Karimganj	0.40	0.84	1.00	0.81	0.74	0.97	0.62	0.77	5.57	0.746	0.252	B
22	Hailakandi	0.46	0.88	0.98	0.81	1.00	0.64	0.57	0.87	6.21	0.776	0.224	B
23	Cachar	0.23	0.93	0.82	0.81	0.87	0.62	0.75	0.00	5.03	0.629	0.371	B

Note : 1. Human Development indicators for the districts are calculated from the values of the eight human development indicators embodied in table 1.

2. While deprivation indices of the districts relating to the indicators $X_1 X_2 X_3 X_4 X_5 X_6 X_7$ and X_8 are calculated by using formula (1), the deprivation index relating to the indicator X_6 (infant mortality per one thousand birth) is calculated by using formula (2)

3. B implies 'backward' and MD implies 'moderately developed'.

Table –13.3

Human Development Indicates in Districts of Assam (by indexing Method)

Sl. No.	District	X_1	X_2	X_3	X_4	X_5	X_6	X_7	X_8	Total development index as P.C. of state average as 100	Average Deprivation Index	Status
1	Dhubri	38.31 (72)	11.95 (110)	0.90 (73)	0.15 (30)	0.37 (77)	0.0078 (92)	63.83 (109)	5878 (86)	549	68.63	B
2	Kokrajhar	40.57 (77)	11.97 (110)	0.76 (62)	0.24 (48)	0.71 (148)	0.0128 (117)	57.35 (98)	5892 (86)	746	93.25	B
3	Bagaigaon	49.06 (93)	11.70 (107)	1.08 (88)	0.24 (178)	0.64 (133)	0.0082 (75)	52.91 (91)	6666 (98)	733	91.63	B
4	Goalpara	46.81 (89)	13.45 (124)	1.27 (103)	0.89 (132)	0.37 (77)	0.0094 (86)	48.37 (83)	5837 (86)	720	90.00	B
5	Barpeta	43.24 (82)	9.49 (87)	1.62 (132)	0.93 (186)	0.43 (90)	0.0099 (91)	40.94 (70)	6534 (96)	834	104.25	R.D.
6	Nalbari	55.95 (106)	9.75 (88)	1.56 (127)	0.59 (118)	0.75 186)	0.0104 (95)	66.23 (113)	5978 (88)	891	111.38	R.D.

(Contd.)

Sl. No.	District	X_1	X_2	X_3	X_4	X_5	X_6	X_7	X_8	Total development index as P.C. of state average as 100	Average Deprivation Index	Status
7	Kamrup	65.04 (123)	7.29 (67)	1.24 (101)	0.54 (108)	0.52 (118)	0.0130 (119)	56.67 (97)	8758 (128)	857	106.38	R.D.
8	Darrang	42.00 (79)	11.00 (101)	1.10 (89)	0.76 (152)	0.49 (102)	0.0090 (83)	52.62 (30)	4740 (69)	765	99.63	B
9	Sonitpur	48.14 (91)	9.41 (87)	1.04 (85)	0.21 (42)	0.44 (92)	0.0130 (119)	70.10 (120)	6031 (88)	724	90.50	B
10	Lakhimpur	58.96 (111)	18.16 (167)	2.67 (217)	0.53 (106)	0.48 (100)	0.0089 (82)	64.72 (111)	7208 (106)	1000	125.00	R.D. (3)
11	Dhemaji	53.84 (102)	19.42 (170)	1.56 (127)	0.62 (124)	0.41 (85)	0.0088 (81)	62.77 (107	6191 (91)	896	112.00	R.D
12	Marigoan	47.99 (91)	16.77 (154)	1.37 (111)	0.31 (62)	0.37 (77)	0.0114 (105)	58.94 (101)	8062 (118)	819	112.00	R.D.
13	Nagaon	54.74 (103)	14.48 (133)	0.94 (70)	0.26 (52)	0.51 (100)	0.0133 (95)	59.17 (100)	9998 (147)	813	101.00	R.D.

(Contd.)

Sl. No.	District	X_1	X_2	X_3	X_4	X_5	X_6	X_7	X_8	Total development index as P.C. of state average as 100	Average Deprivation Index	Status
14	Golaghat	58.54 (111)	11.01 (101)	1.47 (120)	0.72 (144)	0.53 (110)	0.0164 (150)	60.13 (103)	6995 (103)	931	117.63	R.D
15	Jorhat	65.51 (124)	10.59 (98)	2.31 (188)	1.95 (390)	0.62 (129)	0.0244 (224)	69.20 (118)	6496 (95)	1366	170.75	R.D. (1)
16	Sibsagar	64.46 (122)	10.57 (98)	1.65 (134)	0.66 (132)	0.44 (92)	0.0175 (161)	48.42 (83)	9940 (146)	968	121.00	R.D. (4)
17	Dibrugarh	83.35 (110)	12.15 (112)	1.12 (91)	0.38 (76)	0.33 (69)	0.0196 (180)	53.46 (91)	5991 (88)	817	102.13	R.D.
18	Tinsukia	50.28 (95)	9.85 (221)	0.69 (56)	0.20 (40)	0.32 (67)	0.0137 (126)	64.81 (111)	5282 (77)	663	82.88	B
19	Kari Anglong	45.75 (86)	14.22 (131)	0.98 (80)	0.30 (60)	0.81 (1690)	0.0132 (121)	53.41 (91)	6675 (98)	836	104.50	R.D.
20	N.C. Hill	57.76 (109)	33.75 (311)	0.99 (80)	0.66 (132)	0.99 (206)	0.0093 (85)	64.83 (111)	5813 (85)	1119	139.88	R.D. (2)

(Contd.)

Sl. No.	District	X_1	X_2	X_3	X_4	X_5	X_6	X_7	X_8	Total development index as P.C. of state average as 100	Average Deprivation Index	Status
21	Karimganj	54.71 (103)	11.55 (106)	0.58 (47)	0.50 (100)	0.42 (87)	0.0090 (83)	51.92 (89)	6909 (101)	716	89.50	B
22	Hailakandi	53.07 (100)	10.51 (98)	0.62 (50)	0.50 (100)	0.22 (46)	0.0101 (93)	53.48 (91)	5922 (87)	665	83.13	B
23	Cachar	59 (112)	9.12 (84)	0.97 (77)	0.49 (98)	0.32 (67)	0.0133 (122)	48.14 (82)	14060 (206)	848	106.00	R.D.
24	Assam	52.89 (100)	10.56 (100)	1.23 (100)	0.50 (100)	0.48 (100)	0.0109 (100)	58.40 (100)	6816 (100)	800	100.00	

Note:
1. Figure in parentheses refer to the values of indices computed on the basis of state average as 100
2. In respect of infant mortality per one thousand Birth (X_6) we have taken the reciprocal values of X_6 since higher values of X_6 implies lesser human development and consequently higher values of $1/X_6$ will imply higher development.
3. B implies 'backward' & R.D. implies 'relatively developed'.

REFERENCES

Mahbuh-ul-Haq : "Employment and Income Distribution in the 1979s' : A New Perspective", Pakistan Economic and Social Review, June-December, 1971, p.6

United Nation Development Programme : Human Development Report (Delhi; Oxford University Press):

1990 : Concept and Measurement of Human Development

1994 : New Dimensions of Human Development

1996 : Economic Growth and Human Development

1997 : Human Development to Eradicate Poverty

14

HUMAN DEVELOPMENT SCENARIO IN ASSAM

– Hiranmoy Roy

I

Human Development is now-a-days widely used terminology, which reveals the levels of living and quality of life of people in a nation, state or district. Human development differs significantly from Human resource Development and the former is a wider term as it includes all the sections of the society and don't treat human beings simply as factors of production.

The human resource development approach emphasises the need for the development of human capital through education, in-service training, health care, nutrition, housing in order to raise productivity. The human development approach on the other hand, concentrates mainly on the provision for all people the basic means of well-being which inter alia includes food, education and health care.

The policy governing the process of economic development may be explained from two different view points. One is the process of human resource development, that is the 'development of human capital'. The alternative approach is the 'process of enlarging the range of peoples choice' as defined by United Nations Development Programme (UNDP).

Human Resource Development considers human beings as factors of production and seeks to increase their productivity though investment. Increasing productivity is the goal and welfare and levels of living of people are secondary aspects. But in human development approach human beings are not simply considered as factors of production like other factors. More importantly levels of living and well being are emphasized.

Human Development (HD) as well as Human Resource Development (HRD) put man at the centre stage of development process. The concept of Human Development is based on the idea that people are the real wealth of a nation and should therefore be the main beneficiaries of economic development.

HRD uses the capacity and ability acquired by man as means for rapid economic growth of the nation, so that man is treated on par with other inputs. The concept of HD is much broader concept and it considers man as the end of all developmental process and capability or ability as means towards that end. The various facets of HD is captured by a single index called Human Development Index (HDI).

Human Development was defined for the first time by United Nations Development Programme (UNDP) when published its ever first Human Development Report in 1991. Amartya Sen and Mahbub-Ul-Haq through their writings on levels of living popularised the concept and Mahbub-Ul-Haq officially defined the term for UNDP. Human Development captures three indicators namely literacy, life expectancy and per capita income. It was decided that a nation, state or district advanced in these there direction would be considered as having higher human Development and levels of living. Human Development is measured by an index called Human Development Index (HDI). HDI ranges between zero to one.

Mahbub-Ul-Haq stressed on the levels of living in South-

Asia as countries like India, Bangladesh, Pakistan and Nepal are laying far behind the develop countries in terms of levels of living specifically when compared through literacy, life expectancy and per capita income. Amartya Sen cited the examples of China where the achievement of higher levels of living with highest population had set an example for Asian countries. He also advised to learn from Indian states like Kerala and West Bengal as these states with lower state income achieved higher socio economic development and levels of living.

II

In Human Development Report (UNDP) 2003, India ranked 127th out of 170 counties. The first National Human Development Report published by Planning Commission, the National Human Development Report (NHDR-2001). This report ranked different states of India according to HDI. Assam was ranked 14th out of major 15 Indian states in terms of HDI. Economic Survey 2002-03 ranked different North Eastern states (table 14.1). Assam was ranked 26th with an index of 0.34 out of all the states and union territories of India. Mizoram is at most advantageous position and ranked 7th with an index of 0.548. Manipur and Nagaland are relatively better placed as 9th and 11th. Tripura is at 22nd position and Arunachal Pradesh is in most disadvantageous position as ranked 29th. Conditions of Meghalaya is also not good and ranked 24th.

Table 14.1

HDI in North East States of India

States	HDI	Rank
Assam	0.348	26
Arunachal Pradesh	0.328	29
Manipur	0.536	9
Meghalaya	0.365	24
Mizoram	0.548	7
Nagaland	0.486	11
Tripura	0.389	22

Source : Economic Survey 2002-03

The region scores over most other states of India in its relatively high literacy rates. Except Arunachal Pradesh and Meghalaya all other states in the region have literacy rates above the national literacy rates (Sachdeva : 2000). Though literacy rates are higher in the region, Human Development Index is very low (excluding Mizoram). This is due to lower per capita income and poor medical and health services in the region.

III

The ever first Human Development Report of the state, Assam Human Development Report (AHDR : 2003) has been published recently. In this report different districts were ranked according to HDI. The index of twenty-three districts ranges from 0.650 to 0.214. Human Development is higher in most of the east Assam districts. Conditions of west Assam districts are not very good while south Assam districts are relatively better compared to west Assam districts. These generalizations are true except few districts as revealed from the table 14.2.

Table 14.2

HDI of Assam (District wise)

Districts	HDI	Rank	Districts	HDI	Rank
Jorhat	0.650	1	Sonitpur	0.357	13
Kamrup	0.574	2	Nogaon	0.356	14
Golaghat	0.540	3	Kokrajhar	0.354	15
Karbianglong	0.494	4	Nalbari	0.343	16
Morigaon	0.494	5	Lakhimpur	0.337	17
Dibrugarh	0.483	6	Goalpara	0.308	18
Sibsagar	0.402	7	Karimganj	0.301	19
Cachar	0.402	8	Dhemaji	0.277	20
Barpeta	0.369	9	Bongaigaon	0.263	21
Tinsukia	0.377	10	Darrang	0.259	22
Hailakandi	0.363	11	Dhubri	0.214	23
N.C. Hills	0.363	12			

Source: Assam Human Development Report-2003.

Lower levels of human development in North Eastern states may be due to low per capita income and urban bias in medical services. NSDP of the states are far below than the other states of India. The low level of economic activity and dependence on central dole responsible for lower human development in the region. Again health care facilities are mostly available in urban areas offered by both private and public institutions. In rural areas where more than 70 per cent of people live such facilities are scarce.

Publication of Human Development Reports and emphasis on human development has brought a change in development thinking, which must be incorporated in development plan of states and districts and efforts must be made to improve the quality of life of the downtrodden and disadvantageous sections.

REFERENCES

Deptt. of Planning, Govt. of Assam (2003): *Assam Human Development Report.*

Economic Survey (2002-2003) : Govt. of India.

Haq, Mahbub Ul (1996) : *Reflections on Human Development,* Oxford University Press, New Delhi.

Planning Commission (2001) : *National Human Development Report,* New Delhi.

Sachdeva, Gulson (2000) : *Economy of the North East,* Konark Publishers Pvt. Ltd., New Delhi.

15

SELF HELP GROUP– BANK INTERLINKAGES: THE EMERGING PATTERNS IN NORTH EAST INDIA

– Abhijit Sarkar

Introduction

Human Resource Development is the most important issue all over the world, especially in the less developed countries. Human Resource Development plays a very prominent role in the economic development of a country. Underdeveloped human resources are considered to be obstacles to economic development of a country. Some indicators of human resource development are education, health, housing, drinking water etc. But one important factor for human resource development that requires attention is availability of micro credit. The micro credit has succeeded in reducing poverty to a great extent. One modern innovation of micro credit is advancing of credit to the Self Help Groups by formal credit institutions through SHG-Bank linkage.

Review of Literature

Various study reports and the NSS report reveal that the growth rate (elasticity) of employment in India is gradually declining along with rapid population growth. The scope of wage employment or salaried employment mainly in the public sector is gradually shrinking. In the private sector due to rapid mechanization and technological advancement, the need for labour force is diminishing. The consequence is the increase in the volume of unemployed mass (around 26 cores according to NSS 55th Round) that, in turn, leads to poverty.

In this condition, the human resource development naturally suffers a setback. One way to reduce the unemployment problem is to shift the unemployed mass towards self-employment. Now self-employment requires both physical capital and financial capital, the later one being the most important for a sustainable self-employment programme.

The availability of finance is the main problem for the unemployed or the poor. This can be explained from two perspectives-one from the perspectives of type of credit seeker (rich and poor) and another from the demand and supply sides of credit.

a) If one categorizes the population into rich and poor, then it is well established that the rich has better financial stability, the poor having less access to credit facilities. The rich has comparatively better and easy access to credit while the poor are devoied of such accent since they have no asset to credit as they do not have collateral to advance.

b) Again the demand and supply side of credit may be considered. Even after a rapid expansion of banking network since nationalization of banks and introduction of Regional Rural Bank concept, a high percentage of poor people continue to remain outside the purview of the formal credit system that may be due to the problems both from the demand and supply sides of credit. In the supply side, the formal credit institutions find the cost of transaction for lending money to the poor to be high enough. There may also be chance of non-repayment of loans due to improper utilization of advanced money. Moreover from the perspective of the banks, it is not viable to meet the small, emergent and frequent needs of the poor. From the demand side, the poor feel it a hassle to walk a long distance to the banks foregoing the day's work in the field. Moreover the poor try to avoid the paper works and inordinate delay in getting loans. Thus there is always a gap between the demand and supply of credit.

Based on the various studies by different committees and different institutions, it is revealed that the main step that is required for proverty alleviation and for encouraging the people towards self-employment is people's participation through community based organizations. The habit of savings should also be created among the poor for ensuring smooth repayment of the loans. All these observations led to the introduction of SHG-Bank Linkage in February 1992–a bridge for linking the borrower and the lender in a cost effective and sustainable manner–a milestone for the human resource development in the country.

Present Study

The objective of this chapter is to make a comparative study of the flow of credit to the SHGs in the north-eastern states vis-a-vis India as a whole. This is mainly based on the secondary data collected mainly from NABARD, Agartala Regional Office.

SHG concept

A Self Help Group is a small group of poor people, preferably of about twenty, more or less from the same socio-economic class. Each of the group members normally saves at a regular basis a certain sum of money. The savings are kept with the bank in the name of SHG. The members develop self – confidence and mutual confidence after a sufficient period of lending of savings among themselves, in order to access large credit at low rate of interest from banks at a later stage. The default rate of repayment is almost nil due to group pressure for repayment. In short, the members of SHG come together for the following reasons (Basu and Jindal : 2000).

- To save small amount of money regularly

- To mutually contribute to a common fund
- To have collective decision making
- To meet their emergency needs
- To solve problems through mutual discussion
- To have collateral free loans with terms decided by the group
- **SHG –Bank Linkage**

SHG Bank Linkage is a strategy for promoting 'relationship banking', for promoting financial transactions between the formal credit institutions and the SHGs, with the Non Government Organization (NGOs) performing a great role as intermediary.

The banks act as financer whereas the NGOs act as mobilizer of funds and capacity builder of the poor. The linkage models predominantly used are represented through flow charts 15.1–15.4

FLOW CHART 15.1
SHG-BANK LINKAGE MODEL

Direct Linkage Model

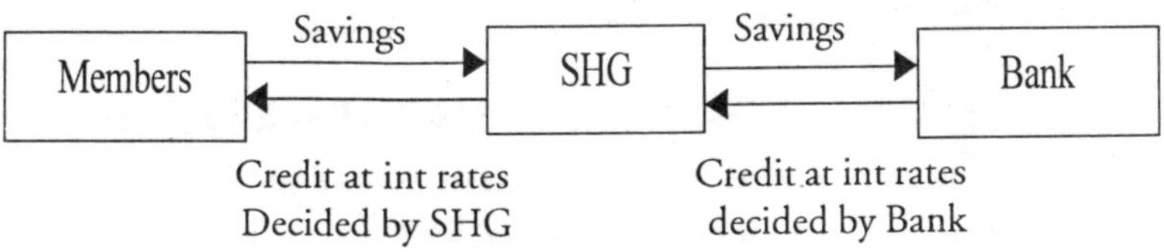

FLOW CHART 15.2
SHG–BANK DIRECT LINKAGE MODEL (MODIFIED):I

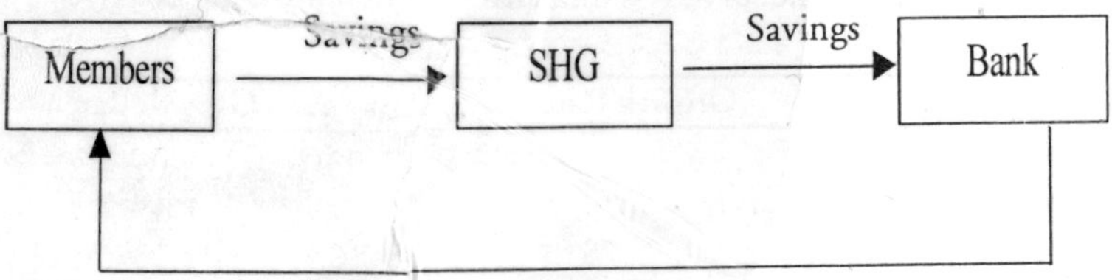

Interest rate on credit is decided by Bank depending upon the amount of loan

FLOW CHART 15.3
SHG–DIRECT LINKAGE MODEL (MODIFIED): II

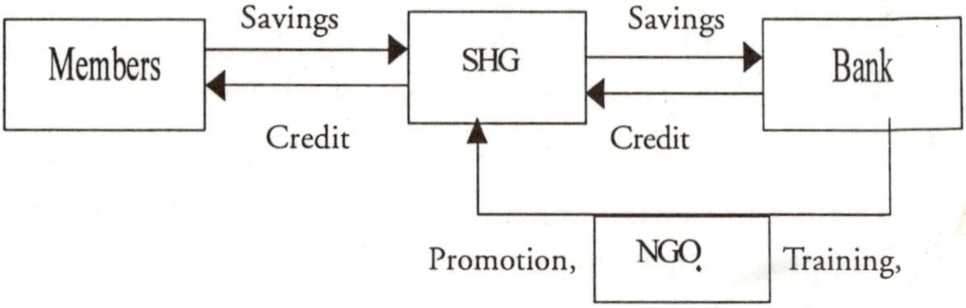

FLOW CHART 15.4
SHG–BANK INDIRECT LINKAGE MODEL

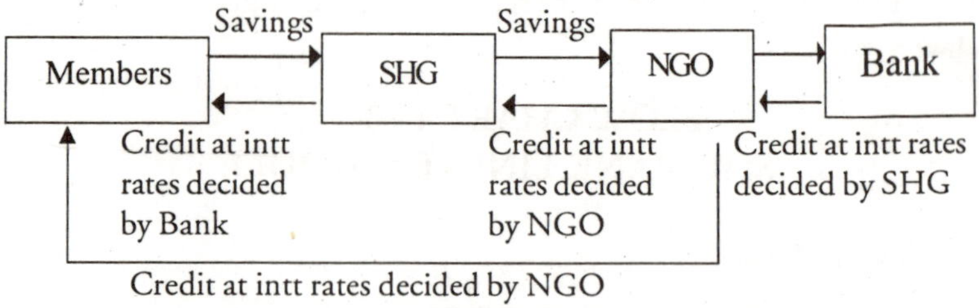

- **Regional Comparative Profile of SHG –Bank Linkage**

The total number of SHGs financed by banks till 31st March 2003 raised upto 7,17,360 from 4,61,478 in 2001-02. The progress of SHG-Bank linkage in the Indian context can be made clear from Table 15.1.

Table 15.1
Progress of SHG-Bank linkage in the India

Year	Cumulative no. of SHGs financed		Cumulative Bank Loan(Rs million)	
	Numbers	Growth Rate	Amount	Growth Rate
1999-2000	1,14,775	-	1,930	-
2000-2001	2,63,825	1.29	4,809	1.49
2001-2002	4,61,478	0.75	10,263	1.13
2002-2003	7,17,360	0.55	20,487	0:99

Source: Progress of SHG-Bank linkage in India 2002-2003, NABARD

From Table 15.1 it can be easily seen that, though there is increase in the absolute number of SHGs linked with banks, yet the growth rate of SHG financed is gradually declining The growth rate that was 1.29 in 2000-01 declined to mere 0.55 in 2002-03. Similar is the case with the amount of bank loans advanced to these SHGs. Thus the growth rate of advance of loans had shown a declining trend though there is rise in its absolute value. The pattern of growth in SHG-Bank linkage in the north-eastern states can be compared with the Indian scenario.

Table 15.2
Trend in the cumulative growth in SHGs linked to Banks

Year	North-eastern Region		India	
	Number of SHGs	Growth Rate	Number of SHGs	Growth Rate
Mar 1999	93	-	32,995	-
Mar 2000	196	1.11	1,14,775	2.47
Mar 2001	477	1.43	2,63,825	1.30
Mar 2002	1490	2.12	4,61,478	0.75
Mar 2003	4069	1.73	7,17,360	0.55

Source: Progress of SHG-Bank linkage in India 2002-2003, NABARD

Most interestingly, the growth rate of number of SHG-bank linkage had shown a falling trend but that in the north-eastern states, it is upward rising with a slight fall in 2002-03. However it is to be noted that this positive growth of SHG- bank linkage in north-eastern region is made possible by the joint efforts of NABARD, Commercial Banks, Regional Rural Banks, Cooperative Banks , NGOs and most importantly by the SHGs (table 15.2).

Let us now look into the regional spread of physical and financial progress in SHG-Bank linkage in the country (upto March 2003) with special reference to the north-eastern states (Table 15.3).

Table 15.3: Regional spread of Physical and Financial progress in SHG-Bank linkage

Region/State	Cumulative no. SHGs provided with bank loan upto 31/03/2002	Cumulative no. SHGs provided with bank loan upto 31/03/2003	Cumulative bank loans upto 31/03/2002 (Rs in million)	Cumulative bank loans upto 31/03/2003 (Rs in million)
North East @	1,490(0.32)#	4,069 (0.56)	25.40 (0.25)	60.32 (0.29)
Assam	1,024	3,477	13.65	45.50
Meghalaya	179	179	5.79	5.79
Tripura	7	104	0.33	0.98
Sikkim	23	24	0.44	0.66
Manipur	134	162	2.61	4.81
Arunachal P.	108	108	2.00	2.00
Nagaland	15	15	0.58	0.58
Northern	19,321 (4.18)	34,923 (4.87)	373.11 (3.64)	771.29 (3.77
Eastern	45,892 (9.94)	90,893 (11.37)	467.51 (4.55)	1204.34 (5.87)
Central	48,181 (10.45)	81,583 (11.37)	569.11 (5.54)	1447.46 (7.07)
Western	29,318 (6.36)	42,180 (5.87)	515.12 (5.03)	869.12 (4.25)
Southern	3,17,276 (68.75)	4,63,712 (64.65)	8313.14 (80.99)	16134.24 (78.75)
India	461478 (100)	717360 (100)	10263.39 (100)	20486.77 (100)

Source: Progress of SHG-Bank linkage in India 20002-2003, NABARD

Figures within bracket indicate percentage to total; @ Data on Mizoram is not available

Compared to other regions of the country, the percentage of SHGs linked with banks in the northeast is almost negligible. Similarly the share of bank loan advanced in the northeast region to SHGs in the country is also very low. Among the northeast states Assam, Meghalaya and Manipur have shown some progress.

The credit to the SHGs are advanced by the Commercial Banks, Regional Rural Banks and Cooperatives with refinance from NABARD.

The Regional Rural Banks play the dominant role in loan advances to SHGs in the Northern, Northeast, Eastern and Central regions of the country whereas in the Western and Southern regions the leading role is played by commercial banks.

Some key issues which need attention are as follows:

1. There should be flexibility in the number of members under SHG. Usually 10 to 20 members can form an SHG. The lower restriction may be lowered further.
2. Normally from one family only one person can become a member of an SHG. This number may be raised to 2 or 3 so that the family can become economically better off.
3. Mixed groups consisting of male and female are not preferred. This restriction may be withdrawn. There are some activities in which the efforts of both males and females are required and which may ensure more productive outcome.
4. The rules of SHG should differ according to socio-economic conditions, e.g. rules of formation of SHG and also SHG-Bank linkage should be different for tribal -non tribal and also for urban-rural people.
5. The rules and SHG-Bank linkage should be made as simple as possible not only for the benefits of the banks but also for SHGs.

Table 15.4: Agency-wise cumulative loan advances to SHGs (up to March 2003)

Region/State	Commercial Banks		Regional RuralBanks		Cooperative banks		Total	
	No. of	Bank Loan	No. of	Bank loan	No. of	Bank loan	No. of	Bank loan
North east @	640	15.93	3386	43.54	43	0.85	4069	60.32
Assam	282	2.82	3158	41.91	37	0.77	3477	45.50
Manipur	162	4.81	-	-	-	-	162	4.81
Meghalaya	62	5.48	117	0.31	-	-	179	5.79
Sikkim	24	0.66	-	-	-	-	24	0.66
Tripura	2	0.16	96	0.74	6	0.88	104	0.98
Nagaland	-	-	15	0.58	-	-	150	0.58
Arunachal	108	2.00	-	-	-	-	108	2.00
Northern	13404	259.57	14512	331.19	7007	180.53	34923	771.29
Eastern	27573	424.69	41352	564.25	21968	215.4	90893	1204.34
Central	27550	441.29	49067	936.85	4966	69.32	81583	1447.46
Western	23718	516.00	13459	256.95	5003	96.17	42180	869.12
Southern	268176	9837.61	155564	5139.02	39972	1157.61	463712	16134.24
India	361061	11495.09	277340	7271.8	78959	1719.88	717360	20486.77

Source: Progress of SHG-Bank linkage in India 2002-2003, NABARD

@ Data on Mizoram is not available

6. Awareness programmes about SHG formation and SHG-Bank linkage should be organized frequently (especially in the north-eastern states).
7. The implementing staff of the banks should be well trained and they must have adequate knowledge about the locality and the people.

Conclusion

This chapter outlines a bird's eye view on the trend in the flow of credit to the SHGs through the SHG-Bank linkage system. There is further scope of research in this area. The introduction of the concept of Self-Help Group can be denoted as the starting of a new chapter in the field of self-employment and also as an efficient tool of Human Resource Development. The SHG-Bank linkage added momentum to the employment generating programmes. The inclusions of 7,17,360 SHGs under bank finance up to March 31,2003 is a great achievement. It is worth mentioning that 11.6 million poor families comprising of 58 million poor people are now under the purview of SHG-Bank linkage. But it cannot be ignored that the progress rate of such linkage is now slowing down. The north-eastern states have got very little attention in the whole process. Efforts should be made to form of more and more SHGs in the north-east and they should be covered under the bank finance, keeping in mind the locational, topographical and economical backwardness of the region.

REFERENCES

Basu K. and Jindal K. (ed) (2000): Microfinance- Emerging Challenges, Tata Mc Graw Hill,

Misra P. and Pari V.K.(2003): Human Resource Development , Indian Economy, Himalaya Publishing House Progress of SHG-Bank linkage in India 2000-2003, NABARD.

INDEX